Essential Writing, Communication and Narrative Skills for Medical Scientists Before and After the COVID Era

Gian Carlo Di Renzo
Editor

Essential Writing, Communication and Narrative Skills for Medical Scientists Before and After the COVID Era

Springer

Editor
Gian Carlo Di Renzo
Department of Obstetrics and Gynecology
Centre of Perinatal and Reproductive Medicine, University of Perugia
Perugia
Italy

ISBN 978-3-030-84956-6   ISBN 978-3-030-84954-2 (eBook)
https://doi.org/10.1007/978-3-030-84954-2

This Springer imprint is published by the registered company Springer Nature Switzerland AG
The registered company address is: Gewerbestrasse 11, 6330 Cham, Switzerland

Preface

A lecturer should appear easy and collected, undaunted and unconcerned
Lecturers which really teach will never be popular; lecturers which are popular will never really teach

Michael Faraday, "Advice to lecturers" 1848

When the COVID-19 pandemic occurred, all the main communication systems of medical research have undergone an epochal change. Many online journals and magazines have tried to publish inherent works of this specific problem as soon and as fast as possible, soliciting and preferring them to others, thus changing the system of free acceptance of scientific works once. Moreover, the way to communicate these works has no longer occurred through standard scientific congresses but with other systems, websites/streaming and webinars or virtual conferences.

Now there is something systematic missing, which foresees that this may last in the future, in the post COVID-19 era (AC): the communication system of the medical sciences will be different from now on. There will be far fewer classical-style conferences like the ones so popular before COVID-19 outbreak (BC) but there will be more webinars, in streaming and virtual or so-called hybrid conferences. In any case, these should change their format to fit with the new requests and modern advances and attendees' fears and doubts which will persists for years.

The book idea is based on the legacy left by Michael Faraday, the famous American chemist, who sensed how communicating what happens in science can make the difference between the success and failure of the research itself. In order to maintain the success in medical communication, we should therefore adapt to new styles and be master of the new systems of media communication.

This new book fits well in this period, creating a bridge between those who do research, how it is communicated, what are the "traditional" communication methods and what is all the necessary background to communicate with new tools.

The volume approach is multidisciplinary and written by top experts in the field of communication and education. It will be a useful tool for scientists in this moment of epochal change in medical communication.

It looks that from now on to communicate research, all scientists will "pop op on camera"!

Hope you enjoy and track useful information for organising your research, your papers and your congresses or courses… AC !

Perugia, Italy Gian Carlo Di Renzo

Contents

1 **The Island of Research (Do Not Block the Path of Enquiry)** 1
Gian Carlo Di Renzo, Valentina Tosto, and Valentina Tsibizova

2 **Big Data, Metanalysis and Sistematic Reviews: The Jungle of Statistics** 19
Naomi Cano-Ibáñez, Marta Maes-Carballo, and Khalid Saeed Khan

3 **Personal Branding and Social Customer Relationship Management in Science, Nurturing Research?** 37
Ricardo Cunha Lopes

4 **Essentials on Writing a Paper for a Peer Reviewed Journal** 45
Marta Maes-Carballo, Khalid Saeed Khan, and Naomi Cano-Ibáñez

5 **The Value of the Websites and Online Journals: The Modern Science** 59
David Bloomer

6 **The Website Construction: The Door to Open Communication** 77
Filippo Gruni

7 **Ways to Implement Scientific Communication in the COVID-19 Era and Beyond** 89
Gian Carlo Di Renzo, Valentina Tosto, Valentina Tsibizova, Khalid Saeed Khan, and Shehnoor Azhar

8 **The "Traditional" Meetings and Congresses** 99
Jonathan P. Wyatt

9 **The New Ways to Communicate Your Research: Webinars and Beyond** 113
Alexandre Manuel Henriques Almeida

10 The Virtual Theater: The Lure, the Title, the Scene, the Backstage, and the Space 125
Andrew Juurinen

11 Just in Time Medical Storytelling 149
Roger Carl Schank

Epilogue 159

About the Authors

Alexandre Almeida He is coordinator of the European Projects Department, including responsibility for setting strategy, identifying opportunities for business, management team and department budget and preparation of proposals for the Horizon 2020 Framework Programmes and other European Programmes to support research, innovation and technological development. He has more than 12 years' experience in the coordination of European proposals setup and managing projects.

Shehnoor Azhar He is a dentist by profession and a Fulbright scholar. He is enrolled as the doctoral researcher at the Department of Clinical Medicine and Public Health, University of Granada, Spain. He teaches occupational health at the University of Health Sciences in Lahore, Pakistan, and has been actively engaged in Phase III clinical trials aimed at finding effective COVID treatments and vaccines.

David G. T. Bloomer He is the president of the Global Library of Woman Medicine, now the Education Platform of FIGO. He is a lawyer (from Oxford University) and later founder partner in a publishing group (Parthenon). In 2009, he founded the largest website dealing with woman health in the world. He is one of the major experts in website building and an honorary fellow of the Royal College of Obstetricians and Gynaecologists.

Naomi Cano-Ibáñez She holds a PhD in clinical medicine and public health. She is a distinguished investigator (Postdoctoral position) at the Faculty of Medicine, University of Córdoba (Spain), where she develops teaching and research tasks related to nutritional epidemiology and advanced statistical analysis. She is an expert on public health and community nutrition. She is a part-time lecturer of public health at the University of Granada (Spain).

Marta Maes Carballo She is a breast cancer specialist and surgeon in the Complexo Hospitalario Universitario de Ourense, Spain, and researcher at the Department of Preventive Medicine and Public Health, Faculty of Medicine,

University of Granada, Spain. Her researches focus on breast cancer management, shared decision-making, and health care quality.

Filippo Gruni Expert in Digital Marketing e Strategist. web designer, developer, visual designer, marketing specialist and content specialist. As founder of Lotrèk, he manages the commercial initiatives, the communication strategy, and the direction of the brand. He is digital strategist of the Start-Up Teeser (Getapp srl) and president of the Young Accountants.

Andrew Juurinen He is director of Marketing at Honeycomb Worldwide Inc., which operates Xtalks.com—a website focused on delivering and marketing webinars and other multimedia for professionals in the life sciences. In this role, he is responsible for overseeing the production and marketing of webinars and other multimedia content in coordination with many leading scientists and brands in the pharma, biotech and medical device arena and is a recognized expert in this field. Andrew obtained his BSc from the University of Waterloo and an MSc in biochemistry from the University of Victoria, Canada.

Khalid Saeed Khan He is a distinguished investigator at the University of Granada, Spain. He is former editor in chief of the British Journal of Obstetrics and Gynaecology and associate editor of BMJ Evidence-Based Medicine. He is professor of public health and preventive medicine and an expert on trials and meta-analysis. He is recently appointed to the prestigious role of COMSTECH Distinguished Scholar.

Ricardo Lopes He is head of Digital and Marketing Strategy at Loba.cx; he manages the digital communication strategy and the direction of several renowned brands. He is also professor at IPAM - The Marketing School, leading a course unit at the Global Marketing Master's Degree. Ricardo is a Ph.D. researcher in digital media at Universidade do Porto (FEUP), where he is developing a taxonomy of digital human behavior.

Gian Carlo Di Renzo He is Professor of Obstetrics and Gynecology, coordinator of the Centre of Perinatal and Reproductive Medicine, University of Perugia and Director of the PREIS School of Firenze, Italy. He is a professor at the Department of Obstetrics and Gynecology at the I M Sechenov First State University of Moscow (Russia). He is the founder and editor in chief, Journal of Maternal Fetal and Neonatal Medicine (UK), and the honorary editor in chief, Maternal Fetal Medicine (China).

Roger Carl Schank He is an American artificial intelligence theorist. He was a professor at Carnegie Mellon University of Texas. He is a cognitive psychologist, educational reformer, and entrepreneur, and he has a very big experience on narrative science and medicine. He wrote several assays on the conceptual representation for a computer-oriented semantics and many other books on this area. In 2012, Dr

Schank founded XTOL (Experiential Training Online) which designs learning by doing experiential short courses for use by universities, corporation, and professional organizations.

Valentina Tsibizova She is an obstetrician-gynecologist, a maternal-fetal medicine specialist, and chief fetal surgeon, Research Laboratory of Operative Gynecology, Institute of Perinatology and Pediatrics at Almazov National Research Centre and at Prenatal Regional Genetic Centre Leningradskaya Hospital, St Petersburg, Russia. She obtained her international doctorate (PhD) at the IE Sechenov First State University of Moscow. She is editorial board member of the Journal of Maternal Fetal and Neonatal Medicine (Taylor and Francis, London) and of Pediatric Cardiology (Warsaw). Since 2020, she is an International Advisory Board member of the Global Library for Women Medicine (GLOWM) endorsed by FIGO.

Valentina Tosto She is an obstetrician-gynecologist, maternal-fetal medicine specialist, and PhD student in translational medicine at the University of Perugia, Italy. She is a consultant at the Department of Obstetrics and Gynecology, Gaslini Pediatric Institute, Genova, Italy. She received a diploma of proficiency from the International PREIS School (Firenze, Italy); she has extensively published in Maternal, Fetal & Neonatal Medicine and in international textbooks.

Jonathan Wyatt He is a specialist in emergency medicine and in forensic medicine and author of the best-selling textbook "Oxford Handbook of Emergency Medicine," which sold more the 130,000 copy worldwide; he is involved in the University of Exeter Medical School and has a biggest experience in organizing meetings, courses, and congresses.

Chapter 1
The Island of Research (Do Not Block the Path of Enquiry)

Gian Carlo Di Renzo, Valentina Tosto, and Valentina Tsibizova

1.1 Introduction

The world of scientific research is articulated and involved many figures, and it is largely influenced by many dynamics.

The original and profound nature of a research should be giving contribution to improve knowledge and even having an impact (hopefully a positive impact) on the human life.

As a researcher (or a scientist, as you want), you are expected to produce and share your research results with others in several forms. Timing and ways of doing research are profoundly changed in the last decades, according to evolving contexts in each field.

In essence, research is performed to enlighten our understanding of a contemporary issue relevant to the needs of society. To accomplish this, a researcher should begin a work for a novel topic based on *curiosity, creativity, critical thinking, and logic*. This leads to the fundamental key elements of the research

G. C. Di Renzo (✉)
Department of Obstetrics and Gynecology, Centre of Perinatal and Reproductive Medicine, University of Perugia, Perugia, Italy

Department of Obstetrics and Gynecology, IM Sechenov First State University, Moscow, Russia
e-mail: giancarlo.direnzo@unipg.it

V. Tosto
Department of Obstetrics and Gynecology, Centre of Perinatal and Reproductive Medicine, University of Perugia, Perugia, Italy

V. Tsibizova
Almazov National Medical Research Centre, Health Ministry of Russian Federation, Saint Petersburg, Russia

G. C. Di Renzo (ed.), *Essential Writing, Communication and Narrative Skills for Medical Scientists Before and After the COVID Era*,
https://doi.org/10.1007/978-3-030-84954-2_1

endeavour: question, objective, hypothesis, experimental tools to test the hypothesis, methodology-design, data analysis, results, and conclusions. When correctly performed, research should produce and spread new knowledge in the scientific community. Important cornerstones of good research are the well-formulated project protocol or proposal that is well executed, analysed, discussed, and concluded [1].

In this essay, I would like to share considerations and opinions about the world of research, how it changed during decades and what are its main keystones, moving by the unique representation of Ernest Harburg in his original poster "The Island of research", that in the 1960s caught some essential findings on the way of doing research and nowadays is still really actual (Fig. 1.1).

The scientific research stimulates debates, different opinions and sometimes controversies amongst all involved figures. Clinical-scientific purposes are strictly related and dependent on specific interests as described below. Experts tried to educate researchers in the critical steps involved in the development of a scientific idea, its successful execution, and eventual publication. Studies have investigated the impacts of research on society, bringing to bear a fresh approach informed by a more holistic understanding of the research enterprise as a complex, versatile, and dynamic system.

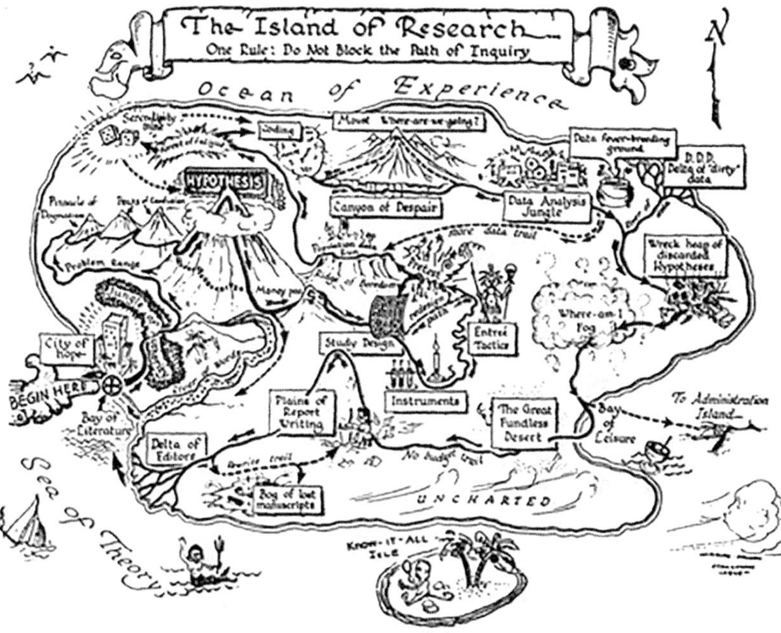

Fig. 1.1 "The Island of research. One rule: do not block the path of inquiry" by Ernest Harburg, 1966

1.2 The Island of Research: A Charming and Adventure Tour

"The Island of research. One rule: do not block the path of inquiry" is a illustration by Ernest Harburg (from the University of Michigan. Box 1.1), prepared with Elaine Stallman and drawn by William Brudon. It was first published in *The American Scientist 54:470, 1966* and called "Research Map" [2]. Later the illustration was used as a cover in a book, *The Science Game* by Neil Mck Agnew and Sandra W. Pake published in 1978.

The fascinating map has aroused great curiosity amongst researchers for its disarming truthfulness. Is not a charming image?

The complexity underlying the world of research emerges from this image. The reading of the opera may be not immediate: the first impact could result strong, but paying attention and using a critical point of view the observer can start an "original tour" amongst the essential key points of the island of research. There are both references to good and negative aspects that characterized clinical research. Is there a provocative intent or only an "aseptic allegorical" illustration in this image? ... Probably the answer to these questions is to be left in the eyes of the beholder!

A simple transcript of map features in line with the interpretations given during the years is:

Point of start (qualities of a good researcher: curiosity, passion, conventional and anti-conventional thinking, logic) → Sea of Theory = Sea of Literature (what we already know) → City of Hope (where ideas are born and the researchers believe in) → Jungle of Authority → Problem Range → Pinnacle of Dogmatism → Peaks of Confusion → HYPOTHESIS → River of Words [→ Money Pass] → Study Design → Instruments → Redesign path → Pretest → Ridge of Boredom → Population data Run → Forrest of Fatigue [→ Never give up, Serendipity mine] → Ocean of Experience [→ Where-are-we-going?] → Canyon of Despair → Data Analysis Jungle [→ too data, technologies and softwares, quality of analysis] → River of Data → also "dirty" data → Wreck heap of discarded Hypotheses [Bay of Leisure → To Administration Island] → The Great Fundless Desert → No budget Trail → Plains of Report Writing [→ Rewrite Trail → Bog of lost manuscripts] → Delta of Editors (many influencing factors) → Bay of Literature (again here ... source of comparison, confirmation or denial, new insights for future) → **ARRIVAL? ...**

... Are we sure that at the end of this adventurous journey there is an arrival? The figure does not show it clearly; it leaves this aspect in suspense, according to the principle of research and its never-ending history. Each research is a journey that has a goal, but not a definitive arrival!

Box 1.1 Ernest Harburg's Profile

- Senior Research Scientist, Emeritus, Department of Epidemiology and Department of Psychology, University of Michigan;
- Founding President and Board Member, The Yip Harburg Foundation;
- Member, Glocca Morra Music Publishing LLC.
- College of the City of New York B.S.S. 1951 History.
- University of Wisconsin, Madison M.A. 1956 Cultural Anthropology.
- The University of Michigan, Ann Arbor Ph.D. 1962 Social Psychology.
- Dr. Harburg's research interests and scholarly publications with a host of collaborators have covered a wide range of topics, including interpersonal conflict, urban life and mental health, rheumatoid arthritis, residential mobility, and correlates of smoking.
- He is best known for his long-term programmatic empirical studies of various correlates and determinants of blood pressure – a series of biological variables, racial, ethnic, and heredity variables, work status and satisfaction, age, personality traits, modes of coping, behavioural patterns and for his more recent work on intra-familial transmission of patterns of alcohol usage.

1.3 Mapping out the Process for Scientific Research

> The practical results do not matter. What counts is the free and disinterested disinterest of the genius of man.
>
> ("The roots of heaven", Romain Gary, 1956)

1.4 Principles of Technical Aspects

Without going in too details, this paragraph describes the technical principles on which clinical research usually moves.

Research is both *theoretical* and *empirical*. It is theoretical because the starting point of scientific research is the conceptualization of a research topic and development of a research question and hypothesis. Research is empirical/practical because all of the planned studies involve a series of rules, observations, measurements, and analyses of data that are all based on proper experimental design [1, 3–10].

Overall, a scientific research development should include several main steps:

- *Define the idea* and the research questions-purposes (the keystone of the entire scientific enterprise. The idea on which a research project is built should be novel, appropriate to achieve within the existing conditions and useful to the medical community and society at large).

- *Literature review* ("the research in the research"; know the state of knowledges in the area of specific topic of interest; it is the process of examining published sources of information, databases, and search engines).
- *Define design and methodology* of the research, consider available sources to carry on.
- D*ata collection* (related with type of research. Several sources and/or modality of collection available now).
- *Statistical analysis* (the process to refer/choose and use sophisticated statistic softwares and other specific networks of data analysis. Modern technologies have greatly improved this research step: large databases available, easier and faster data analysis).
- D*iscuss and draw conclusions* (the process of observation and comparison of study results with already known evidence; analyse and discuss why).
- *Communicate the results* (researchers do not only "do" science but also "write" science to share the evidence, to eventually apply useful results in the clinical practice, to give new insights for future perspectives and further researches).

1.5 Past and Current Trends: Is There a Shift in the Focus?

Great things are not accomplished by those who yield to trends and fads and popular opinion

("On the road", Jack Kerouac, 1957)

Change may be frightening, but it results usually necessary...

Undoubtedly, in the last decades, purposes and interests in scientific research are changed according to the progress of a global system. In the past, the scenario in which scientific research moved was different. Sometimes experts underlined that in the past, the researcher's enthusiasm for a new idea and hypothesis was dominant and the leading element in a context where often sources were less. On the contrary, nowadays research is often blamed for receiving pressure by industry and policy interests. Moreover, it sometimes moves from ideas and projects that arise from specific purposes, not only clinical but also related with personal objectives (career path), the prestige of a department or a country, the economic-financial interests, losing that sense of original and ancient purity, and that high profile of scientific quality. Debates and controversies regard ethical-unethical behaviours, personal/career purposes, research promotion pathways, industries interests/interferences, level of quality of trials, and control systems. As in any field of life, it is necessary to contextualize and recognize the inevitability of progress and its good and bad consequences. Therefore, there is probably a part of truth in the criticisms and debates, but surely the profound high-quality profiles of researchers and their work still survive.

Undoubtedly, clinical trials have been fundamental for understanding disease pathways and in fostering the development of novel treatments (pharmacological therapies, devices, and tools) in medicine. One important issue in this field is how they continue to change over time. From the first recorded trial of legumes in biblical times to the first randomized controlled of trial of streptomycin in 1946, the history of clinical trial covers a wide variety of challenges: scientific, ethical, and regulatory.

Some developments in the clinical research enterprise arised from since World War II. Moreover, a recent study analysing clinical trials in psychiatry over the past 60 years showed substantial changes in the use of statistical methods in the reporting of abstracts and results, as well as increased use in recent trials of informed consent, washout periods, the intention-to-treat approach, and parametric tests [11]. Many of these changes have been shaped by historical events. Main examples, the development of ethical guidelines, have been marked by three milestones: the Nuremberg Code [12] made voluntary consent mandatory for clinical research; the Declaration of Helsinki [13] codified the ethical principles for human experimental research; and the infamous Tuskegee Syphilis Study [12] led to the Belmont Report, which increased protection for human research subjects and defined informed consent in different research settings. Another important historical event that has shaped clinical research is the issue of adverse effects associated with novel interventions. One of the landmark examples is the use of thalidomide, which resulted in unexpected harm to the foetus. Here, the development of study phases (phases I, II, III, and IV) and additional pre-clinical studies has greatly increased the safety of new drugs and devices.

Regulatory changes have also been important in increasing the safety of clinical trials. A heated debate is currently taking place on the use of placebos and the further development of non-inferiority trials. At the same time, some scientists claim that ethics committees are becoming overly bureaucratic and not fulfilling their mission well [14]. Options for balancing the prevention of unethical behaviour with the promotion of research include decreasing the length of research proposals and informed consent forms and giving different review processes according to the risk of the intervention and the benefits to patients. Clinical trial reporting has also been constantly developing to increase transparency in clinical research. One example is the database registry clinicaltrials.gov [15] which has had a significant impact on clinical research. This is also the case for the Consolidated Standards of Reporting Trials (CONSORT) [16, 17], an important effort to improve transparency in reporting randomized controlled trials so that readers can better understand a study's design, methodology, and the validity of its results.

1.6 Some Historical Memories

> The charm of history and its enigmatic lesson consist in the fact that, from age to age, nothing changes and yet everything is completely different.
>
> ("Music at night", Aldous Huxley, 1931)

History is full of anecdotes regarding how the best scientific innovations were born.

The world's first clinical trial we have trace is recorded in the *Book of Daniel* in The Bible [18]. This experiment resembling a clinical trial was not conducted by a medical, but by King Nebuchadnezzar a resourceful military leader [18]. During his rule in Babylon, Nebuchadnezzar ordered his people to eat only meat and drink only wine, a diet he believed would keep them in sound physical condition. But several young men of royal blood, who preferred to eat vegetables, objected. The king allowed these rebels to follow a diet of legumes and water—but only for 10 days. When Nebuchadnezzar's experiment ended, the vegetarians appeared better nourished than the meat-eaters, so the king permitted the legume lovers to continue their diet [18]. This probably was the one of the first times in evolution of human species that an open uncontrolled human experiment guided a decision about public health. Avicenna (1025 AD) in his encyclopaedic *Canon of Medicine* described some rules for the testing of drugs [19]. He suggests that in the clinical trial, a remedy should be used in its natural state in disease without complications. He recommended that two cases of contrary types be studied and that study be made of the time of action and of the reproducibility of the effects. These rules suggest a contemporary approach for clinical trials. However, there seems to be no record of the application of these principles in practice. The first clinical trial of a novel therapy was conducted *accidentally* by the famous surgeon Ambroise Pare in 1537 [18, 20, 21]. In 1537 whilst serving with the Mareschal de Motegni, he was responsible for the treatment of the battlefield wounded soldiers. As the number of wounded was high and the supply of conventional treatment, oil was not adequate to treat all the wounded, he had to resort to unconventional treatment. He described: "... at length my oil lacked and I was constrained to apply in its place a digestive made of yolks of eggs, oil of roses and turpentine. That night I could not sleep at any ease, fearing that by lack of cauterization I would find the wounded upon which I had not used the said oil dead from the poison. I raised myself early to visit them, when beyond my hope I found those to whom I had applied the digestive medicament feeling but little pain, their wounds neither swollen nor inflamed, and having slept through the night. The others to whom I had applied the boiling oil were feverish with much pain and swelling about their wounds. Then I determined never again to burn thus so cruelly the poor wounded by arquebuses". However, it would take another 200 years before a planned controlled trial would be organized. James Lind is considered the first physician to have conducted a controlled clinical trial of the modern era [18, 21], Dr. Lind (1716–1794), whilst working as a surgeon on a ship, was appalled by the high mortality of scurvy amongst the sailors. He planned a comparative trial of the most promising cure for scurvy. Lind described: "... On the 20th of May 1747, I selected twelve patients in the scurvy, on board the Salisbury at sea. Their cases were as similar as I could have them. They all in general had putrid gums, the spots and lassitude, with weakness of the knees. They lay together in one place, being a proper apartment for the sick in the fore-hold; and had one diet common to all, viz. water gruel sweetened with sugar in the morning; fresh mutton-broth often times for dinner; at other times light puddings, boiled biscuit with sugar, etc., and for supper, barley and raisins, rice and currants, sago and wine or the like. Two were ordered each a quart of cyder a day. Two others took twenty-five drops of elixir vitriol three times a day … Two others took two spoonfuls of vinegar three times a day … Two of the worst patients were put on a course of sea-water … Two others had each two oranges and one lemon given them every day … The two remaining patients, took … an electary recommended by a hospital surgeon … The consequence was, that the most sudden and visible good effects were perceived from the use of oranges and lemons; one of those who had taken them, being at the end of six days fit for duty … The other was the best recovered of any in his condition; and … was appointed to attend the rest of the sick. Next to the oranges, I thought the cyder had the best effects …" (Dr James Lind's *Treatise on Scurvy*, published in Edinburgh in 1753).

The first double blind controlled trial (Patulin for common clod; 1943) and the first randomized curative trial (Streptomycin, 1946) later arrived [22]. The latter one derived from the idea of randomization born in 1923. However, the first randomized control trial of streptomycin in pulmonary tuberculosis was carried out in 1946 by MRC of the UK [23, 24]. The MRC Streptomycin in Tuberculosis Trials Committee (1946) was chaired by Sir Geoffrey Marshall, and the statistician was Sir Austin Bradford Hill and Philip Hart, who later directed the MRC's tuberculosis research unit, served as secretary. Marc Daniels, as the "registrar" coordinated the clinicians at the participating hospitals. The trial began in 1947. As the amount of streptomycin available from the USA was limited, it was ethically acceptable for the control subjects to be untreated by the drug – a statistician's dream [23]. This trial was a model of meticulousness in design and implementation, with systematic enrolment criteria and data collection compared with the ad hoc nature of other contemporary research [25].

1.7 Serendipity and Research: "Pleasent Surprise?"

> There will always be serendipity involved in discovery
>
> ("The Guardian" interview, Jeff Bezos, 2002)

As mentioned in previous paragraph, many of the major discoveries in science have been the product of chance observations that were pursued by the curious mind to their plausible and provable explanation. This is right from the past to modern era and explains the concept called "serendipity".

Serendipity is the occurrence of an unplanned fortunate discovery. It is a common occurrence throughout the history of product invention and scientific discovery. It is also seen as a potential design principle for online activities that would present a wide array of information and viewpoints, rather than just re-enforcing a user's opinion. The term was coined by Horace Walpole in 1754. In a letter he wrote to a friend, Walpole explained an unexpected discovery he had made by reference to a Persian fairy tale, *The Three Princes* of Serendip. The princes, he told his correspondent, were "Always making discoveries, by accidents and sagacity, of things which they were not in quest of".

The notion of serendipity is now a common occurrence throughout the history of scientific innovation. In June 2004, a British translation company voted the word to be one of the ten English words hardest to translate. However, due to its sociological use, the word has since been exported into many other languages.

Significant historic events (not only medical) occurring as a result of serendipity include the discovery of the law of buoyancy (Archimedes principle) by the Greek mathematician Archimedes, of the Americas by Christopher Columbus, and of gravity by Sir Isaac Newton.

Memoirs, autobiographies, and Nobel Prizes acceptance speeches revealed the true nature of famous discoveries.

Mendel's peas and, at least apocryphally, Newton's apple come to mind as paradigm shifting observations that respectively opened the fields of genetics and established the laws of gravitation. Fleming's chance observation of the inhibition of bacterial growth in the presence of bread mould ultimately produced the first antibiotic. The unexpected link between the Australia antigen and the hepatitis B virus may be less encompassing than genetics or gravitation, but nonetheless is a classic example of a serendipitous observation pursued to major unexpected payoffs, including the prevention of post-transfusion hepatitis, the development of a vaccine, the prevention of hepatocellular carcinoma, and laying the foundation for the discovery of non-A, non-B hepatitis, and ultimately the hepatitis C virus. Lamotrigine for bipolar disorder, as others psychotropics, chemotherapy drugs, and antibiotics were more recent additional examples of unplanned source derived from unexpected observations. Nowadays each field of research, scientific and not, shows a story of serendipity before receiving concrete clinical confirmations.

Do not forget the rationality thought that scientific research needs … Discoveries require serendipity, but serendipity is not a chance alone! It is a process in which a chance event is seized upon by a creative mind who chooses to pay attention to the event until find a proper application for it. Thus, brilliant minds of successful scientists may have the insight and creativity to recognize a "Eureka!" [26].

The prevalent convention of all scientific writing is to present studies as rationally driven: this is right, but remember to have both conventional and anti-conventional thought, to have a flexible mind and see over the schemes. Research needs to both processes of logical experiments, rational deductions, and intuition and creative acts.

Serendipity is an important theme in medical innovation. There is no reason to think this will change or must change. Things do not necessarily go as planned, but often the results are as important as the original prediction was supposed to be. It will not be clear where we end up until we try and get there.

1.8 Globalization Effect on Clinical Research

> You have no choice but to operate in a world shaped by globalization and the information revolution. There are two options: adapt or die.
>
> ("Fortune", Andy Grove, 1995)

Nowadays, globalization is showing important effects on the conduct of clinical research. Brunoni and Fregni [12] found that more multicentre trials are being conducted. Glickman et al. who discuss the economic benefits of globalization found that clinical trials increasingly occur on a global scale and claim that one-third of trials are now being conducted in developing countries as pharmaceutical and medical device companies have embraced globalization [27, 28]. This clearly raises numerous ethical concerns, including the testing of drugs for wealthy populations in human subjects of developing countries, the exacerbation of economic disparities and exploitation of low-income workers in developing countries, and their exposure to potentially dangerous drugs that could not be approved for testing in developed countries.

Globalization is probably the keystone and driving concept to which many others are linked at the basis of change in the scientific world. It contributed to the change of way of thinking, of planning, and of working.

Scientific research has led to behaviours of global competition for scientific purposes, commercially viable technologies, and other innovations. For many decades, the USA has led the world in science and technology, but nowadays the competition evolves. Discoveries from scientific research have extended our understanding of the physical and natural world, the cosmos, society, and humans – their minds, bodies, and economic and other social interactions. Through these discoveries, science has enabled longer and healthier lives, provided for a better-educated citizenry, enhanced the national economy, and strengthened countries' position in the global economy.

1.9 Research Training Programs

Tell me and I forget, teach me and I may remember, involve me and I learn

("The achievements of the Ru", Xun Kuang "Xunzi, 3rd Century BC)

With this rapidly changing environment and increasingly complex system, the training of clinical researchers becomes ever more critical. One of the topics in clinical research that needs to be addressed is the increasing number of studies that use complex statistical analyses which can be difficult for readers to interpret [29]. Standard clinical research training requires students to be present on site, but this prevents some from participating owing to limited time and funds. One of the more innovative models of training programs for clinical researchers uses the principle of collaborative learning [30, 31], in which participants build and learn by discussing the concepts and ethics of clinical research in a course forum that blends live lectures (via video-conference) with online discussion and small-group work with highly trained teaching assistants [32]. Clinical research training is a relatively new academic field, and curricula in the design and conduct of clinical research have only emerged since the 1980s. The growing complexity of clinical trials and the emergence of evidence-based medicine in the last several decades created great demand for clinicians with knowledge of clinical epidemiology and biostatistics. Amidst alarm bells rung by physician-scientist leaders about the endangered species of clinical researchers, numerous proposals and solutions emerged to address these workforce and educational problems in the 1990s [33]. Di Renzo et al. published a chapter on the way to develop a research project and write a scientific paper with the aim to guide students and researchers in their work [34].

1.10 Scientific Integrity: A Milestone to Preserve

> Be daring, be different, be impractical, be anything that will assert integrity of purpose and imaginative vision against the play-it-safers, the creatures of the commonplace, the slaves of the ordinary.
>
> ("Glass of fashion", Cecil Beaton 1954)

Research operates in a continuous and rapidly changing world. We previously said that change should be welcome with a positive acceptance, even if it often brings debate and critical dynamics. One of this is the scientific integrity, a milestone concept at the basis of the scientific thought and purpose. It depends on a set of foundational expectations that all science should be built upon to maintain trust. Failures of scientific integrity may not be more common now than in the past, but they may be more visible. In the twenty-first century, scientists work in a research environment influenced by globalization, interdisciplinary research projects, team science, and information technologies. As the scientific enterprise evolves, all stakeholders in the scientific community have an ethical obligation to give a high priority on instilling and championing the highest standards of scientific integrity in these new settings and applications [35]. There is currently no universal and shared definition of scientific integrity. Yet an agreed-upon definition of scientific integrity and other key terms is crucial to understanding the boundaries of the principles and best practices. Some agencies' definitions incorporate research integrity as part of scientific integrity, whilst other agencies separate both terms. The Consortium agreed that for the purposes of these principles and best practices, the terms "scientific integrity" [as defined by the US Department of the Interior (DOI—it conserves and manages the Nation's natural resources and cultural heritage for the benefit and enjoyment of the American people, provides scientific and other information about natural resources and natural hazards to address societal challenges and create opportunities for the American people, and honours the Nation's trust responsibilities or special commitments to American Indians, Alaska Natives, and affiliated island communities to help them prosper], "research misconduct" (as defined by the U.S. Federal Research Misconduct Policy), and "detrimental research practices" (as defined by the U.S. National Academies of Sciences, Engineering, and Medicine 2017 report *Fostering Integrity in Research*) would be used in the development of the principles and best practices for scientific integrity [35]. Main definitions of this concept are reported in Table 1.1.

Table 1.1 Definitions [35]

• *Scientific integrity* The US Department of the Interior (DOI) defines scientific integrity as "the condition that occurs when persons… adhere to accepted standards, professional values, and practices of the relevant scientific community… adherence to these standards ensures objectivity, clarity, and reproducibility, and utility of scientific and scholarly activities and assessments and helps prevent bias, fabrication, falsification, plagiarism, outside interference, censorship and inadequate procedural and information security…"
• *Research misconduct* The Federal Research Misconduct Policy sets forth a uniform definition of research misconduct, defined as "fabrication, falsification, or plagiarism in proposing, performing or reviewing research, or in reporting research results. Research misconduct does not include honest error or differences of opinion". Canadian federal research agencies use the term "breach" rather than "research misconduct", in which "breach" is defined as the "failure to comply with any agency policy throughout the life cycle of a research project—From application for funding, to the conduct of the research and the dissemination of research results"
• *Detrimental research practices* The report, *fostering integrity in research*, coined a new term, "detrimental research practice," for instances when researchers "engage in other behaviour [beyond research misconduct] that clearly damages research". When researchers commit detrimental research practices or research misconduct, they "stray from the norms and appropriate practices of science". The consortium supports the use of this new term. A similar term, "questionable research practices", is used in Canada and abroad

A Scientific Integrity Consortium developed a set of recommended principles and best practices that can be used broadly across scientific disciplines as a mechanism for consensus on scientific integrity standards and to better equip scientists to operate in a rapidly changing research environment. The two principles that represent the umbrella under which scientific processes should operate are as follows [35]:

1. Foster a culture of integrity in the scientific process.
2. Evidence-based policy interests may have legitimate roles to play in influencing aspects of the research process, but those roles should not interfere with scientific integrity.

Moreover, the nine best practices for instilling scientific integrity in the implementation of these two overarching principles were defined as follows [35]:

1. Require universal training in robust scientific methods, in the use of appropriate experimental design and statistics, and in responsible research practices for scientists at all levels, with the training content regularly updated and presented by qualified scientists.
2. Strengthen scientific integrity oversight and processes throughout the research continuum with a focus on training in ethics and conduct.
3. Encourage reproducibility of research through transparency.
4. Strive to establish open science as the standard operating procedure throughout the scientific enterprise.

5. Develop and implement educational tools to teach communication skills that uphold scientific integrity.
6. Strive to identify ways to further strengthen the peer review process.
7. Encourage scientific journals to publish unanticipated findings that meet standards of quality and scientific integrity.
8. Seek harmonization and implementation amongst journals of rapid, consistent, and transparent processes for correction and/or retraction of published papers.
9. Design rigorous and comprehensive evaluation criteria that recognize and reward the highest standards of integrity in scientific research.

The concept of scientific integrity is really complex and regards other important milestones in research field, such as fabrication, falsification, destruction of research records, plagiarism, redundant publication or self-plagiarism, invalid authorship, inadequate acknowledgement, mismanagement of conflict of interest, misrepresentation in a grant application or related documents, mismanagement of grants or award funds, breach of agency policies or requirements for certain types of research, and breach of agency peer review processes.

Buckwalter et al. stated that "Science, being a high-stakes enterprise, is based on the ability to produce new and important observations [36]. An academic and/or industry scientific career is dependent on publication, which in turn has an impact on continued employment, promotion, grant support, personal recognition, and competition with other investigators". Presently, there are metrics to evaluate an individual scientist, but they do not fully encompass the spirit and goal of this best practice. One existing way that a researcher's career is evaluated is through the *h*-index, which "attempts to measure both the productivity and citation impact of the publications of a scientist or scholar" and is "based on the set of the scientist's most cited papers and the number of citations that they have received in other publications". There must be community consensus and alignment around the necessity for scientific integrity standards and their content.

1.11 Relationship with Industry and Conflicts of Interest

"Doctors & druggists wash each other's hands"

("Canterbury tales", Geoffrey Chaucer, 1387)

Scientific research and medical practice collaborate with pharmaceutical, medical device, and biotechnology companies to develop products that benefit individual and public health. At the same time, concerns are growing that wide-ranging financial ties to industry may unduly influence professional judgments involving the primary interests and goals of medicine. Such conflicts of interest threaten the integrity of scientific investigations, the objectivity of professional education, the quality of patient care, and the public's trust in medicine. Surveys show the breadth and diversity of relationships between industry and physicians, researchers, and educators in academic and community settings.

Industry shows an important role in research field, both for medical-therapeutic purposes and financial interests. This explains why drug and device companies involved in healthcare circuits develop close interactions with physicians.

A recent interesting paper investigated whether industry-sponsored drug and device studies have more favourable outcomes and differ in risk of bias, compared with studies having other sources of sponsorship. From this, systematic review and meta-analysis resulted that pharmaceutical and device studies sponsored by manufacturing companies have more favourable efficacy results and conclusions than studies sponsored by other sources [37].

Conflicts of interest (COI) are defined as a set of circumstances that creates a risk of professional judgment concerning a primary interest being unduly influenced by a secondary interest [38]. All healthcares are usually involved in these dynamics. For doctors, such conflicts may arise from interactions with pharmaceutical companies, amongst others [39–41]. Moreover, studies have shown that industrial interests may influence physicians' decisions and may thus have negative effects for patients and the healthcare system [42]. Recent surveys have shown that medical students also interact with pharmaceutical companies on a regular basis and feel inadequately prepared for these interactions by their universities [41]. It therefore seems to be reasonable to raise awareness for the effects of COI amongst medical students and residents early on in their training. Other researches underlined the importance of clinical setting in influencing this relationship, such as public practice versus private practice. Overall, many factors can affect the link between industry, medical decision-making, and conflict of interest. In the USA [43], Australia [44], most of the European countries [45], and Japan [46], pharmaceutical companies have been required to publicly report the payments they provide to physicians. In the USA, payment data from pharmaceutical and medical device industries have been available since 2013 through the Open Payments program; the UK has required these data since 2016. Previous studies have suggested that board specialists, medical journal editors, executive board members of professional medical associations, and clinical practice guideline (CPG) authors are critical targets for pharmaceutical payments. All these features aspire to make clear and transparent interactions between industries and healthcare systems [47].

On the light of dualism between advantages and potential risks deriving from relationship between industry, medical attitudes, and conflict of interests, experts provided some useful tips and recommendations [37]:

1. Payments arising from industry-sponsored research should be centralized in institutional funds and not paid directly to researchers.
2. Should be transparency about the source and the purpose of the payment.
3. Company sponsorship of medical societies and their educational events should be kept to a minimum and declared quantitatively in societies' websites and scientific programme brochures.
4. All speakers should declare their conflicts of interest at their scientific meetings. Guideline groups should require all members to declare their financial COI before meeting and exclude or limit those members with COI.

Governmental authorities should not allow continuing medical education credits to those educational events not complying with the above policies. The crucial role of medical journals as "gatekeepers" for identifying "science" must be reaffirmed.

1.12 "One Rule: Do Not Block the Path of Enquiry"

> By way of watching your mind, you will see life beyond a mere set of habits, emotions and beliefs
>
> ("Unbound intelligence", Rajeev Kurapati, 2020)

"One role: do not block the path of enquiry" is part of title that Ernest Harburg gave to his famous illustration. But, what did he mean by this statement? Does it underline a lucid and critical allusion to the way of conducting and doing research?

This sentence resounds as a sort of request that the course of scientific research is not hindered.

We do not know what hindering factors Harburg was referring to. In general, this invitation is addressed to any factor that disturbs the principles on which the scientific research moves, many seen in the previous paragraphs. As previously seen, the journey to the research island is full of inevitable pitfalls, which probably must be part of this course; the researcher must have a brilliant mind capable of transforming pitfalls into opportunities or avoid influencing his way of thinking.

As Kurapati say, looking at your mind you can look at your life in its deepest essence and even beyond. In any historical era, the only rule of science is not "to clip the wings" of those who have curiosity, a critical mind, and passion and believes he can offer a contribution with his conventional and non-conventional thinking!

1.13 Conclusion

Even if we are now in the era of globalization, of ethical changes, of modern industries, and of financial issues, Harburg's allegorical scheme is still actual about 60 years after its creation. The evolution of clinical research traverses a long and fascinating journey, is still on course, and is destined to a "never-ending history". As long as researchers think with a conventional and non-conventional mind and the scientific integrity principle is respected, the essence and high quality of scientific research will be safe.

The "Island of research" is not only a simple illustration, but is a "piece of history" that remind to the beholder that:

> Research is to see what everybody else has seen, and to think what nobody else has thought
>
> ("Bioenergetics", Albert Szent Gyorgyi, 1957)

References

1. Balakumar P, Inamdar MN, Jagadeesh G. The critical steps for successful research: the research proposal and scientific writing: (a report on the pre-conference workshop held in conjunction with the 64(th) annual conference of the Indian pharmaceutical Congress-2012). J Pharmacol Pharmachoter. 2013;4(2):130–8. https://doi.org/10.4103/0976-500X.110895.
2. Harburg E. Research map. Am Sci. 1966;54:470.
3. Jagadeesh G, Murthy S, Gupta YK, et al. Biomedical research—from ideation to publication. 1st ed. Philadelphia: Wolters Kluwer health-Lippincott Williams and Wilkins; 2010.
4. Balakumar P. In: Jagadeesh G, Murthy S, Gupta YK, Prakash A, editors. Biomedical research. From ideation to publication. Philadelphia: Wolters Kluwer health-Lippincott Williams and Wilkins; 2010. p. 212.
5. Balakumar P, Marcus SJ, Jagadeesh G. Navigating your way through online resources for biomedical research. RGUHS J Pharm Sci. 2012;2:5–27.
6. Reisman F. Creative, critical thinking and logic in research. RGUHS J Pharm Sci. 2011;1:97–102.
7. Bartz CC. Getting started with research: ideas to research process. RGUHS J Pharm Sci. 2011;1:176–9.
8. Kuberappa YV, Kumar AH. Knowing the known to understand the unknown-a systematic approach to reviewing the scientific literature. RGUHS J Pharm Sci. 2012;2:1–7.
9. Neville C. Referencing: principles, practice and problems. RGUHS J Pharm Sci. 2012;2:1–8.
10. Balakumar P, Murthy S, Jagadeesh G. The basic concepts of scientific research and communication. Indian J Pharm. 2007;39:303–6.
11. Balakumar P, Jagadeesh G. The basic concepts of scientific research and scientific communication. J Pharmacol Pharmacother. 2012;3:178–82.
12. Brunoni AR, Fregni F. Accelerating response to antidepressant treatment in depression: review and clinical suggestions. Prog Neuropsychopharmacol Biol Psychiatry. 2010;34:437–8. https://doi.org/10.1016/j.pnpbp.2010.01.011.
13. Pressel DM. Nuremberg and Tuskegee: lessons for contemporary American medicine. J Natl Med Assoc. 2003;95:1216–25.
14. WMA Declaration of Helsinki. Ethical principles for medical research involving human subjects.2008. http://www.wma.net.
15. White R. Institutional review board mission creep: the common rule, social science, and the nanny state. Independent Rev. 2007;11:547–64.
16. A service of National Institute of Health. Understanding clinical trials. What is a clinical trial? 2010. http://www.clinicaltrials.gov.
17. Consort statement. 2010. http://www.consort-statement.org.
18. Plint AC, Moher D, Morrison A, et al. Does the CONSORT checklist improve the quality of reports of randomised controlled trials. A systematic review. Med J Aust. 2006;185:263–7.
19. Collier R. Legumes, lemons and streptomycin: a short history of the clinical trial. CMAJ. 2009;180:23–4.
20. Bull JP. A study of the history and principles of clinical therapeutic trials, 1951. MD thesis, University of Cambridge.
21. Twyman R A. A brief history of clinical trials, 2004. The Human Genome. http://genome.wellcome.ac.uk/doc_WTD020948.html.
22. Chalmers I, Milne I, Trohler U, et al. The James Lind library editorial team. The James Lind library: explaining and illustrating the evolution of fair tests of medical treatments. J R Coll Physicians Edinb. 2008;38:259–64.
23. Bhatt A. Evolution of clinical research: a history before and beyond James Lind. Perspect Clin Res. 2019;1(1):6–10.
24. Hart PD. A change in scientific approach: from alternation to randomised allocation in clinical trials in the 1940s. BMJ. 1999;319(7209):572–3.

25. MRC Streptomycin in Tuberculosis Trials Committee. Streptomycin treatment of pulmonary tuberculosis. BMJ. 1948;2:769–83.
26. Yoshioka A. In: Emanuel EJ, Grady C, Crouch RA, Lie RK, Miller FG, Wendler D, editors. The randomized controlled trial of streptomycin in the Oxford textbook of clinical research ethics. Oxford: Oxford University Press; 2008. p. 46–60.
27. Meyers MA. Happy accidents. In: Serendipity in modern medical breaktroughts. New York: Arcade Publishing; 2007.
28. Glickman SW, McHutchison JG, Peterson ED, et al. Ethical and scientific implications of the globalization of clinical research. N Engl J Med. 2009;360:816–23. https://doi.org/10.1056/NEJMsb0803929.
29. Rocha-e-Silva M. Recent trends in Brazilian medical research: an overview. Clinics. 2009;64:1007–13. https://doi.org/10.1590/S1807-59322009001000012.
30. Horton NJ, Switzer SS. Statistical methods in the journal. N Engl J Med. 2005;353:1977–9. https://doi.org/10.1056/NEJM200511033531823.
31. Azeka E, Fregni F. Cardiovascular research: new model of collaborative training program. Arq Bras Cardiol. 2010;95:281–2. https://doi.org/10.1590/S0066-782X2010001300001.
32. Azeka E, Fregni F, Costa Auler JO. The past, present and future in clinical research. Clinics (Sao Paulo). 2011;66(6):931–2.
33. Teo AR. The development of clinical research training: past history and current trends in the United States. Acad Med. 2009;84(4):433–8. https://doi.org/10.1097/ACM.0b013e31819a81c9.
34. Di Renzo GC, Mattei A, Gerli S. Come si scrive un testo scientifico. In: Trattato di Ginecologia e Ostetricia. 2nd ed; 2009.
35. Kretser A, Murphy D, Bertuzzi S, et al. Scientific integrity principles and best practices: recommendations from a scientific integrity consortium. Sci Eng Ethics. 2019;25:327–55.
36. Buckwalter JA, Tolo VT, O'Keefe RJ. How do you know it is true? Integrity in research and publications. J Bone Joint Surg. 2015;97A(e2):1–8.
37. Lundh A, Lexchin J, Mintzes B, et al. Industry sponsorship and research outcome: systematic review with meta-analysis. Intensive Care Med. 2018;44(10):1603–12.
38. Thompson DF. Understanding financial conflicts of interest. New Engl J Med. 1993;329(8):573–6.
39. Zipkin DA, Steinman MA. Interactions between pharmaceutical representatives and doctors in training. A thematic review. J Gen Intern Med. 2005;20(8):777–86.
40. Steinman MA, Shlipak MG, McPhee SJ. Of principles and pens: attitudes and practices of medicine housestaff toward pharmaceutical industry promotions. Am J Med. 2001;110(7):551–7.
41. Lieb K, Koch C. Medical students' attitudes to and contact with the pharmaceutical industry: a survey at eight German university hospitals. Dtsch Arztebl Int. 2013;110(35–36):584–90.
42. Lieb K, Scheurich A. Contact between doctors and the pharmaceutical industry, their perceptions, and the effects on prescribing habits. PLoS One. 2014;9(10):e110130. https://doi.org/10.1371/journal.pone.0110130.
43. Jarvies D, Coombes R, Stahl-Timmins W. Open Payments goes live with pharma to doctor fee data: first analysis. BMJ. 2014;349:g6003.
44. Robertson J, Moynihan R, Walkom E, et al. Mandatory disclosure of pharmaceutical industry-funded events for health professionals. PLoS Med. 2009;6(11):e1000128.
45. European Federation of Pharmaceutical Industries and Associations. Disclosure of payments to HCPs: EFPIA member associations have been working to transpose the EFPIA Disclosure Code. https://www.efpia.eu/relationships-codes/disclosure-of-payments-to-hcps/. Accessed 2018
46. Japan Pharmaceutical Manufacturers Association. Transparency guideline for the relation between corporate activities and medical institutions. http://www.jpma.or.jp/english/policies_guidelines/pdf/transparency_gl_intro.pdf. Accessed 2018.
47. Dodgson SJ. The evolution of clinical trials. J European Med Writers Assoc. 2006;15:20–1.

Chapter 2
Big Data, Metanalysis and Sistematic Reviews: The Jungle of Statistics

Naomi Cano-Ibáñez, Marta Maes-Carballo, and Khalid Saeed Khan

2.1 Introduction

In the fields of health and medical sciences, with the interest focused on diagnosis of human conditions and effectiveness of treatment, there exist a large number of studies carried out in different settings and locations. They have different participants and with different forms of the interventions. They apply various statistics seeking to reveal the best medical option for a health-condition. The main problem related to this synthesis of this evidence is the variability of the results obtained by individual researchers and groups. This makes interpretation of findings and clinical decision-making challenging. Nevertheless, if we assume that the aforementioned variability was something unavoidable and possibly constructive in some

N. Cano-Ibáñez (✉)
Department of Preventive Medicine and Public Health, University of Granada, Granada, Spain

CIBER of Epidemiology and Public Health (CIBERESP), Madrid, Madrid, Spain

Instituto de Investigación Biosanitaria de Granada (ibs.GRANADA), Granada, Spain
e-mail: ncaiba@ugr.es

M. Maes-Carballo
Department of Preventive Medicine and Public Health, University of Granada, Granada, Spain

Department of General Surgery, Complexo Hospitalario de Ourense, Ourense, Spain

K. S. Khan
Department of Preventive Medicine and Public Health, University of Granada, Granada, Spain

CIBER of Epidemiology and Public Health (CIBERESP), Madrid, Madrid, Spain

G. C. Di Renzo (ed.), *Essential Writing, Communication and Narrative Skills for Medical Scientists Before and After the COVID Era*,
https://doi.org/10.1007/978-3-030-84954-2_2

circumstances, then we could synthesize the available information and draw conclusions about the questions asked in evidence-based medicine.

Currently, applied science has the systematic review (SR) as one of the main tools to address the discrepancies generated by the variability of published results. SR is a scientific investigation that comprises an exhaustive, protocolled, and explicit evaluation of the literature based on a clear research question, an explicit methodology, a critical appraisal using relevant tools, and an objective summary of the evidence related to the research topic [1–3]. A key point that should be considered is that a narrative review or a commentary or an editorial or an opinion is not a SR. Note that, unlike SR, such reviews do not use a systematic and explicit methodology to summarize the evidence. Table 2.1 shows the main differences between narrative (non-systematic) reviews and SRs.

A statistical tool, frequently used to summarize the evidence numerically, is the meta-analysis (MA). MA is a technique that combines the results of individual studies to synthesize their results and give an overall estimate. MA is appropriately used by reviewers after they have performed the initial steps of SR searching the literature and extracting data. If the data found primarily is clear, complete, and homogeneous, there are good grounds for applying MA. Frequently, SR is confused with MA. Although there exist conceptual similarities, they are not the same thing. The SR methodically gathers all the available evidence with established eligibility criteria, with a clear objective of answering a specific question. Its methods are explicit so that biases are minimized. The above done, MA statistical technique can then be used to combine the results of individual studies to synthesize their results and generate a single overall estimate. So, SR encompasses the overall scientific process, and MA may or may not be a part of a well-conducted SR. However, MA carried out without an SR would not have a leg to stand on in the absence of systematic searches and quality assessments.

SR and MA are essential scientific instruments for synthesizing available scientific information, increasing the understanding of the findings of individual studies, and identifying areas of gap where more research is necessary. Furthermore, they are indispensable for evidence-based healthcare being useful not only for medical decision-making, but also for policy management related to health [4, 5]. They also underpin guidelines and recommendations. However, conducting a quality systematic review is not an easy task. This chapter aims to present the conceptual bases for

Table 2.1 Main differences between narrative reviews and systematic reviews

Domain	Narrative review	Systematic review
Research question	Unstructured	Structured, with participants, interventions and outcomes identified a priori
Search strategy	Not detailed, not systematic	Detailed and systematic
Study selection	Neither specified nor detailed	Inclusion and exclusion criteria specified in a research protocol
Assessment of study quality	Not aplicable	Assessed by specific tools for capturing risk of bias, validity, reliability etc. using for example GRADE/AMSTAR scales

conducting and interpreting a SR/MA emphasizing key points during their execution through an exemplar review.

2.2 "Big" Data, Meta-Analysis, and Systematic Reviews

SRs and MAs typically synthesize published information related to a specific health topic, guiding healthcare decision while exposing the variability of primary studies. Although SRs collate data, in the globalization era, there are electronic methods to achieve data in large amount, namely, "Big" data. These datasets allow the analysis of data from millions of patients to identify associations between exposures and health outcomes. Such registries are usually established to collect data first, and then research methods are applied to extract results. The benefits of "Big" data have been purported to underpin personalized medicine, as they assess risks and predict outcomes [6, 7], but there is more to healthcare than merely observations made passively about what happened in the course of illness in the past. This would help but will not directly facilitate decision-making in health. The latter requires prospective studies that examine the effects of health policies, via experimental or randomized designs. SRs provide a tool to collate their findings to directly facilitate decision-making. Large datasets, in theory, offer consistent data, an assumption that ought to be tested concerning data quality in each project because patient's clinical records from which "Big" data are derived tend to be unstructured and difficult to read, and some ethical considerations should also be taken into account. Acknowledging the complementarity offered by "Big" data, this chapter will now continue to give more information on SRs.

2.3 Systematic Review Example: Health Effects of Physician-Patient Language Discordance

Imagine just for a moment that you are a political health advisor who must give input into the assignment of that budget of a hospital that serves a large migrant population. You know that migrants have restrictive legal status and socioeconomic difficulties. You have read that language differences between healthcare providers and migrant patients are also recognized as a major global healthcare barrier [8]. However, the evidence of the negative effect of language discordance on healthcare provision is patchy. It may be associated with medication non-compliance, adverse drug events, and underuse of preventative care [9, 10]. Interpreters may play a role in addressing language discordance [11], but this intervention is associated with shortcomings including longer waiting times, increased consultation duration, and financial burden [12]. And you are not sure if focusing on this issue is necessary, or it would be better to allocate the money to other more pressing aspects of healthcare. In order to base your advice on facts, you decided to explore effects across a wider range of healthcare domains among migrants while focusing attention on objective clinical outcomes. Congratulations! You have decided to employ a scientific method. The best option to answer your question is to perform a robust SR.

The first step in carrying out a SR is to design a protocol that includes information about the review methods. It comprises of the research question, the inclusion and exclusion criteria for the selection of studies, and the search strategy with an explicit methodology that will combine various types of search terms to use in different searching databases. This protocol can be peer-reviewed. The protocol should be prospectively registered, e.g., in a database entitled PROSPERO (http://www.crd.york.ac.uk/prospero/). It will provide a public record of planned review methods with a unique ID number. Prepare your prospective registration or review protocol with the need to comply with PRISMA Statement [13] in mind, which you will do well to deploy in writing your review manuscript for publication. Patient and public engagement in protocol development gaining momentum so as to increase the relevance of reviews [14]. PRISMA-P, a checklist for writing review protocols, is also available. To clarify how to perform a quality SR in the above example, we briefly summarize the five steps that you will have to follow based on a paper previously published by Khan et al. [2].

2.3.1 Research Question

The first step is to formulate the research question. Using a published review, [15] the free-form question in the example described above could be: *Is physician-patient language concordance associated with improvements in health outcomes?* To undertake a review, the question must be explicit and structured. It should include the following key components: *participants, intervention or exposure, comparison, outcomes, and study designs* [16].

- *Participants*: Physicians and patients.
- *Exposure*: Physician-patient language concordance.
- *Comparison:* Physician-patient language discordance.
- *Outcomes:* Objective health outcomes, including cancer screening rates, serum HBA1c levels, postoperative length of stay, and blood pressure measurements.
- *Study designs:* Comparative studies with an observational design that examine the outcomes in both groups, one with language concordance and the other without.

2.3.2 Search Strategy and Study Selection

2.3.2.1 Search Strategy

As in any research study, the presence of errors in data collection can invalidate the results of a SR and MA. This step is essential to minimize random error (by capturing a large proportion of the studies ever done) and bias (by capturing a representative sample of the high-quality studies ever done). Firstly, reviewers should develop clear inclusion and exclusion criteria attending to the review question. In addition, it may be pragmatic to narrow down the search results, but applying language restrictions and date of publication may have a limiting effect on the review. Once the impact of the restrictions applied by the selection criteria have been understood, the next stage is to look for the primary studies. Usually, for feasibility reasons, it seems reasonable to include only the studies published in scientific journals, considering that these having passed a peer review process. It is however not necessary that they are more reliable than Master or Doctoral theses which have also undergone a formal assessment. The main search strategy is the use of electronic databases such as MEDLINE (PubMed), Web of Science, SCOPUS, or EMBASE. The identification of potentially eligible articles is usually carried out, for ease of operability, by examining titles and abstracts and with the help of a reference management software. However, each database has its own structure and uses some indexing criteria and keywords more or less specific. For example, in MEDLINE, the specific index of a controlled vocabulary is called MeSH (Medical Subject Headings). Only well-designed search term combinations can provide relevant information for the review.

Following our example, a literature search was carried out across four bibliographic databases, PubMed, Psychinfo, Web of Science, and EMBASE, in June 2020. We did not apply limits to publication date or article language. In order to achieve an optimal search strategy, the following indexing terms, word variants, and free text terms were applied. In PubMed the MeSH-terms combined in the search strategy were: [“Language discordance” OR “Language concordance” OR “language prof*” OR “interprofessional] AND language” [“health outcomes” OR “clinical outcomes” “diabet*“OR “hyperten*” OR “cardiovasc*” OR “psych*” OR“mental health” OR “physical health”] AND [“doctor” OR “physician” OR “clinician”] AND [“patient”]. A manual search, reviewing the reference lists of relevant reviews and primary studies, was also conducted. Endnote bibliographic citation management software was used to pool all the citations that the search yielded. First, we removed all the duplicates.

2.3.2.2 Study Selection

Once we have carried out the search, the databases will throw at us citations of scientific articles related to the review question. At this point, if a few citations are found, there are two possible alternative explanations. One is that the review question proposed has not been previously studied, and the other is that our search term combination construction was not correct. Perhaps this latter option more commonly materializes. In this case, we can reconstruct the search, which gets better with every iteration.

When the correct search has been implemented, the databases used will generate the correct results. Based on the titles and abstracts identified, a first screening of the potential eligible articles can now be performed applying the pre-defined inclusion and exclusion criteria which were prospectively registered with a well-defined protocol. This screening should be undertaken, ideally, by two-independent reviewers, and, if there are any doubts, the full-text article should be reviewed by both independently too before reaching consensus. However, it is common that discrepancies between reviewers exist despite the review of the full article. In this case, a third reviewer (usually senior and with expertise in the field of research) is appointed to arbitrate over the discrepancies generated.

Once completed, the study selection process has to be reported in an orderly way, indicating the articles identified in each phase, as well as those eliminated and the causes of their elimination. A flow-diagram is the best option to do this task as shown in Fig. 2.1. Following our example, the manuscript stated: Two reviewers (give reviewer's initials) independently screened the titles and abstracts and reviewed the full texts for study selection. Articles were initially screened by title and article and were included if they [1] were observational studies, [2] included an exposure group of patients that were identified as language concordant or

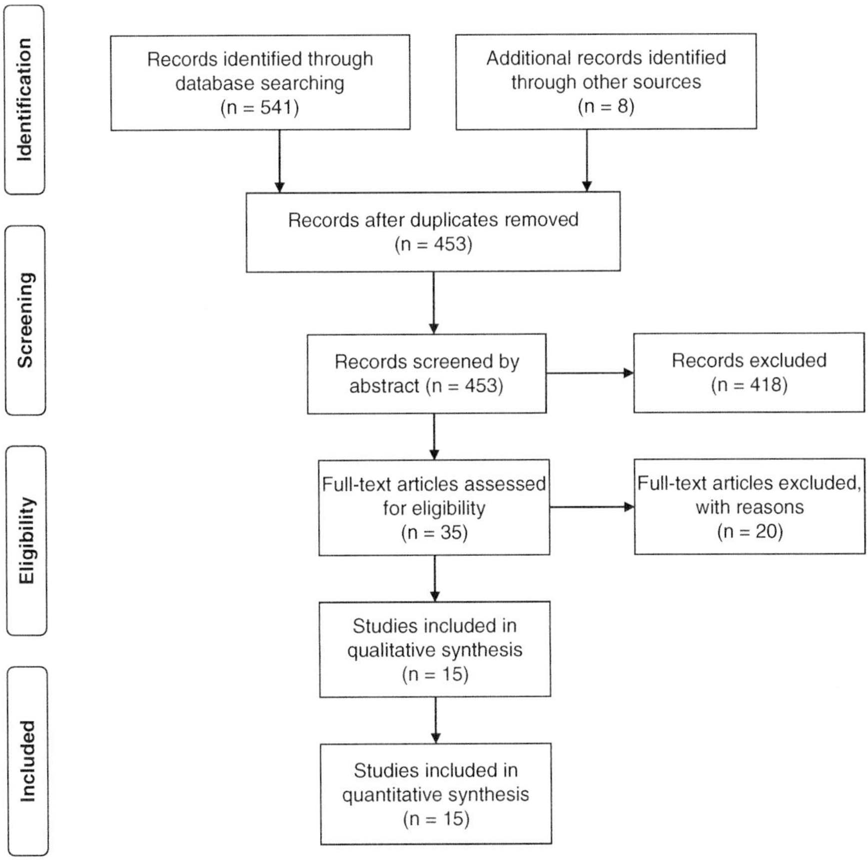

Fig. 2.1 Flow-diagram of study selection (adapted from [15])

discordant with their physicians, [3] identified an association between language discordance and patient health outcomes, and [4] health outcomes observed were objective health measurements, such as cancer screening rates, serum HBA1c levels, postoperative length of stay or blood pressure measurements. Articles that solely included self-reported measures of health outcomes or other forms of subjective outcome measures, such as patient satisfaction of care, patient experience, or medical comprehension were excluded. Articles that only included the use of interpreters and failed to explore physician-patient language concordance specifically were also excluded. Qualitative studies, reports, and grey literature were excluded. As shown in Fig. 2.1, the SR search yielded 541 citations. An additional eight articles were identified through searching reference lists of relevant studies. After removal of 96 duplicates, 451 articles remained for title and abstract screening. After exclusion of 418 articles that did not meet the selection criteria, 35 studies were carried forward for full text review and assessed for eligibility. Fifteen out of the 35 studies were eligible, from which data on study characteristics and main findings was extracted.

2.3.3 *Assessment of the Quality of Studies Included in the Synthesis*

The methodological quality of the studies included in an SR is fundamental in order to assess the risk of bias (internal validity) and to implement evidence-based healthcare in an optimal way using the best available evidence. Selected studies should be subjected to a quality assessment by the use of general critical appraisal guides and design-based quality checklists (Table 2.2). There is a plethora of such tools and instruments (Table 2.2 only gives a very brief overview of tools for reporting quality), but with a little attention, you won't get lost, and it will be possible to find relevant items for quality assessment in your review.

An adequate study design is a key marker of quality; thus a randomized study will be better than an observational one for the evaluation of effectiveness as it reduces selection bias both for known and unknown and measured and unmeasured baseline variables. However, randomized studies are not always possible depending

Table 2.2 Types of tools to assess the quality of published studies

Name of the tool	Kind of study-design
STROBE	Observational studies
CONSORT	Randomized studies
PRISMA	Systematic review and meta-analysis
AMSTAR	Systematic review (randomized primary studies)
NOS	Systematic review (non-randomized primary studies)

on the research question. Thus, SRs that synthesized and compare studies of any design are fundamental to evidence-based practice. Basically, the studies included could exaggerate or underestimate the "true" effect of exposure. This deviation from the truth is known as bias. The main types of biases that may be present in an SR are selection bias, related to the process of obtaining similar comparison groups at baseline; performance bias, related to the process of obtaining similar comparison groups with respect to co-interventions after the inception of the cohort; loss or attrition bias, related to participant or data losses linked to follow-up in primary studies; detection bias, related to systematic differences between comparison groups in the assessment of outcomes; and publication bias, related to missing out studies of small sizes with negative findings. Thus, methodological considerations should be addressed as a part of the review protocol.

Following the example of how the language concordance review took into account the risk of bias among selected studies: "The reviewers independently extracted data and assessed the selected study quality. The risk of bias of each study was assessed using the modified Newcastle-Ottawa Scale (NOS) [17] which addresses three aspects of quality: [1] *Selection*: representativeness of the exposed participants to language discordant care, selection of the non-exposed participants and ascertainment of exposure to language discordant care, [2] *Comparability*: confounders and study design, and [3] *Outcome*: assessment of health outcome, adequate retention of the cohort (%) and follow-up period (years) [17]. All 15 studies were assessed for quality using the modified Newcastle-Ottawa Scale. Ten studies were of good quality, four studies were of fair quality and one study was of poor quality, with positive, negative, or no differences in health outcomes for the language discordance compared to the language concordance group." An example dummy table of quality assessment of primary studies is shown in Table 2.3.

The instruments used to assess the quality of SRs are diverse depending on the review question and related methods. Their choice for new reviewers can be confusing. The most commonly applicable quality assessment tool is AMSTAR [18] (Assessment of multiple systematic reviews) which is used for investigating the methodological quality of published SRs. PRISMA [19] (Preferred Reporting Items for Systematic reviews and Meta-analysis) is an evidence-based minimum set of items for reporting in SR and MA. Finally, GRADE [20] (Grading of Recommendations, Assessment, Development, and Evaluations) is a tool for grading the certainty of the evidence collated in an SR, particularly when used to make recommendations in guidelines [21, 22]. These tools will be used in the interpreting of findings.

2.3.4 Data Synthesis

The data extraction from each included study in a SR should be done by the two reviewers, independently. It is important to note that the selected information to be extracted from primary studies should be included in the review protocol. Usually,

Table 2.3 Items to include in quality assessment of primary studies in a systematic review

Author	Selection of studies				Comparability	Outcomes			Quality score
	Representativeness of exposed cohort	Selection of non-exposed cohort	Ascertainment of exposure	Outcome not at start of Study	Comparability of cohorts	Assessment of outcome	Length of Follow up	Adequacy of follow up	
Manson (1988)	Not truly representative of asthmatic patients and the sample size was small	Yes	Patient language status from chart notes or estated by their physicians	Yes	Adjusted by age, gender, pay-status, disease severity	Electronic medical record	Yes	>40%	Good

the data extraction includes information about authors, year and place of publication, participants, exposures, and design of the study; information about outcomes in form of 2x2 tables and statistical measures (odds ratio, relative risk, confidence intervals, etc.); and information about study quality. Data from individual studies should be collated in a systematic way as shown in dummy tables (Tables 2.4 and 2.5), and then statistical methods can be used to summarize these data if appropriate. In an MA, the most common way of presenting the data is through a graph known as a forest plot or effects diagram. In this graph, the results of each study are represented by the effect using a square and a horizontal line (95% confidence interval). The summary measure of effect and its 95% confidence interval is captured in a diamond. Such graphs also help to examine heterogeneity visually even when MA is not performed.

The association between language concordance and health outcomes was examined in 15 studies. From our example: "The following information was obtained from the articles for analysis: first author, publication year, study locations, study design, sample size, population, type of objective health outcome(s) studied, participants' race and/or ethnicity, languages documented, the effect of language concordance/discordance, comparison groups, and main findings. Compared to concordance, eight studies (53%) showed a significant negative association between language discordance and at least one measure of clinical outcome amongst study participants. Five studies (33%) found no significant association between language discordance and the main clinical outcome. And two studies (13%) found a positive association between language discordance and clinical outcomes." This information can be summarized graphically (Fig. 2.2). This form of "vote" counting is not ideal, but it may be the only suitable method in heterogeneous reviews. The "vote" counting is used to compare the number of studies with positive results vs. the number of studies with negative results. The vote counting is useful to assess whether there is evidence about the effect we wish to measure and it should take into account study quality. "Vote" counting should not be carried out subjectively, but rather it should directly address the initial question about the effect on outcomes we wish to measure [23].

2.3.5 *Interpretation of the Findings*

The final step is to objectively perform the interpretation of the SR findings. This part must include a discussion on the limitations of the review. In the language concordance example, the focus was on the health effects of physician-patient language concordance. Based on the low quality of available studies, caution is needed in the interpretation of findings (Fig. 2.2). The effect of language concordance in improving health outcomes merits consideration. Although you may think that after carrying out such extensive work, the strength of the recommendation is low. This is because your research question cannot be answered confidently, given the study quality. The SR has given you all available information and allowed you to know the

Table 2.4 Items to be included in the synthesis of the characteristics of primary studies

Author	Location	Study design	Sample size	Language(s)	Patients	Race/ ethnicity	Intervention	Health outcomes
Manson (1988)	USA	Retrospective cohort study	96	Spanish; English	Adult Spanish-speaking population with asthma, seen from July 1979 to March 1987	Hispanic	Physician-patient LC vs LD	Serum levels of theophylline; ER visits for asthma, follow-up appointments

Table 2.5 Items to include to synthetize results of studies included in the systematic review

Primary author, publication date, location	Outcomes	Measures	Language discordance (LD) vs. language concordance (LC)	Relative risk (RR) / odds ratio (OR) /mean/ prevalence	95% confidence intervals (CI)/ interquartile range (IQR)	P value
Manson 1988, United States	Medication adherence to asthma inhalers	Non-therapeutic serum theophylline levels (10–20 mg/dl)	LD = 59% LC = 50%	OR = 1.72	CI: 0.69–4.30	0.24
	Emergency room (ER) use	Number of ER attendance	LD = 48% LC = 55%	OR = 2.07		0.12
	Hospital admissions	Number of hospital admissions	LD = 26% LC = 32%			
	Miss a medical appointment	Non-medical attendance (<8 office visits)		OR = 1.66	CI: 0.86–3.20	0.13

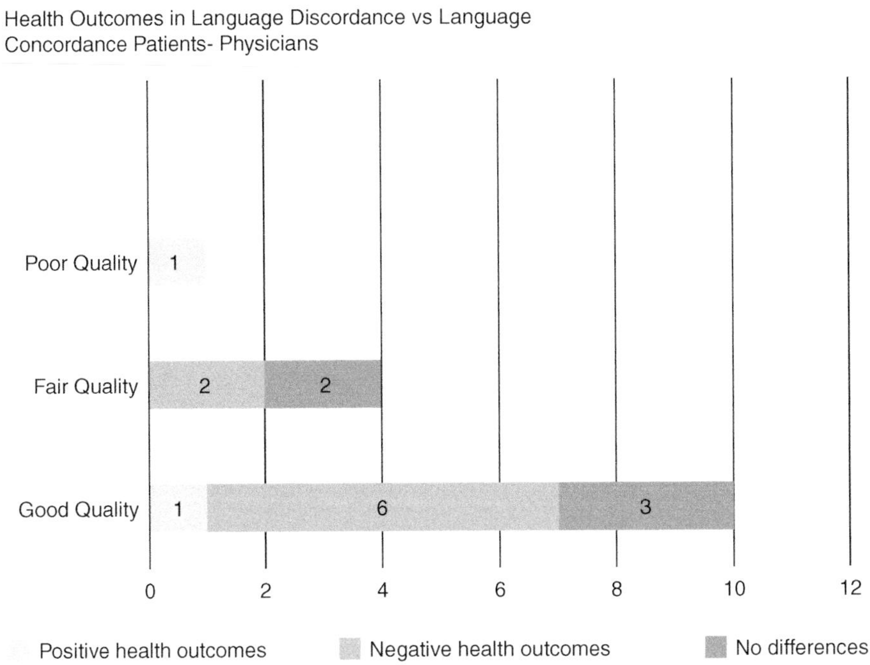

Fig. 2.2 Graphic representation of the quality of the studies through "vote" counting positive, negative, or no differences in health results for the language discordance group compared to the language concordance group

facts about the balance between beneficial and harmful effects of language concordance in migrant's health. Whatever the opinions on this matter, you are able to reassure all parties based on facts. This information can be usefully deployed in your budgetary decision-making and you may even fund a high-quality study to be undertaken in your hospital.

2.4 Guidelines and Shared Decision-Making

The promotion of high-quality healthcare has become a priority in recent years [24]. Despite the fact that a large part of the published work that does not meet quality criteria (as in our exemplar review above) to be considered scientifically valid [25], a more scientific approach can allow health systems to provide a better quality of care and more efficient use of resources [26]. To help in this work, evidence-based statements are developed for standardizing medical interventions and improving healthcare quality as clinical practice guidelines (CPGs). CPGs can be defined as "statements that include recommendations intended to optimize patient care that is informed by a SR of evidence and an assessment of the benefits and harms of alternative care options" [27].

SRs should be used in CPGs to systematically identify, assess, and summarize the ongoing state of management on a clinical topic. These often demand methodological adaptation and innovation so as not to lose out on quality. So, CPGs should all follow a rigorous methodological approach fitting criterion for an SR [28]. However, SRs to develop an evidence synthesis to summarize in CPGs are arduous and time-consuming, which delays deportation of researching into practice. A key feature of the last step of SRs for CPGs is to produce GRADE tables for determining strengths of recommendations [29, 30]. These delays can be associated with a loss of benefits for the patient [31] basing healthcare in outdated CPGs [32] and decreasing their quality [33, 34]. Artificial intelligence could accelerate the transmission of individual research studies into evidence synthesis to concurrently improve the quality of CPGs for guiding healthcare [35].

Shared decision-making is a cornerstone in the attainment of high-quality evidence-based care, and it should be routinely included in CPGs [33]. It gains real importance when different options with similar potential are able to reach very diverse decisions considering patients´ values, beliefs, and preferences [36, 37]. It has been demonstrated that shared decision-making increases the satisfaction of the patient [37], decreases malpractice claims [38], and improves cost-effectiveness [37]. It is a legal obligation in developed countries [39–41], and it is strongly promoted by medical associations [42–44]. However, nowadays, there are still a big amount of barriers in its implementation [45–49], and its implementation in practice is still scarce [50, 51]. SRs need to present their findings in a way that shared decision-making is supported. To achieve this, patient and public engagement in SRs and CPGs is a necessary step.

Many strategies have been proposed for the practical enforcement of shared decision-making [36, 48, 52–55]. One of the models suggests encouraging patients to decide their own care goals that doctors would transform into a diagnostic or treatment project [48, 52]. Another three-step proposal focuses on selecting a choice, describing options, and exploring patients´ preferences [36]. The shared decision-making process is helped by some tools such as option grids and other decision aids [53, 54]. All these efforts require underpinning SRs. Evaluating the shared decision-making as a quality indicator and incentivizing professionals who use shared decision-making can be useful to facilitate implementation [55].

The important subject of shared decision-making should be adequately covered in SRs. There are just a few SRs [33, 56–64] on the topic. All of them highlighted the poor information available. This lack of knowledge is a known barrier for shared decision-making implementation and leaves a large scope for improvement in this area. Therefore, it is necessary to carry out more SRs and MAs with shared decision-making as the final output.

2.5 Rapid Reviews in Times of COVID-19 Pandemic

The pandemic of the coronavirus disease 2019 (COVID-19) has caused infection in 42.8 M cases worldwide and has killed more than 1.15 M people around the world by the end of October 2020 [65]. Its containment is becoming difficult due to the long incubation period with the quick transmission. Nowadays, despite the great efforts that health authorities around the world are making, the lack of knowledge about this new disease is causing concern. Public health measures and infection control are imperatively required to prevent the spread of the virus. Although the Internet allows access to information quickly and easily, on occasions, it can also cause misinformation in the general population. The public has to be well educated, and researchers have to train themselves to engage the public. The collection and summary of the information with a high level of evidence are vital. This is where SRs and MAs are essential as they provide a comprehensive clinical resume of all the available data from high-quality research studies relevant to the epidemiology, demographics, hospital tendencies and consequences, medical signs and symptoms, and diagnostic and treatment methods of COVID-19 [66].

Reviewers are conscious that the current methods of a systematic review are not rapid enough for a pandemic so there is an increased interest in finding ways to accelerate knowledge improvement. Artificial intelligence could be useful in this field as it could accelerate the synthesis of evidence from individual research studies, solving difficult problems in the automation of systematic reviews, and thus allowing a more rapid improvement of the quality of healthcare in the future [35].

2.6 Misuse and Abuse of the SR/MA

Despite the multiple benefits that SRs present, as we mentioned before, these is a serious risk that some SRs could be misleading, useless, or even harmful when methods and data are mishandled, intentionally or unintentionally. One key problem is that health practitioners, while required to train and maintain licensure for practice and clinical trials, need no training, certification, ethical approval or regulatory control for undertaking SRs and MAs. Ready availability of databases and softwares allows for easy experimentation and packaging of findings in apparent SRs. Literally any 'Tom, Dick and Harry" can engage in SRs. The only recourse some quality control lies with editors and peer-reviewers. But, sadly, just as authors don't, they don't either need to undergo any training, certification, competence assessment, or regulatory control for evaluating SRs and MAs prior to publication. As SR/MA tend to yield more citations, journal editors have a tendency to accept them more readily than primary studies so as to use them as a means to boost their impact factor. This allows many wolves to slip into the public domain in sheep's clothing. Even in organized reviewing conglomerates such as Cochrane Collaboration, Campbell Collaboration, and BEME, the checks and balances to ensure quality can slip. Ultimately, the responsibility lies with the reader to acquire competence in critical appraisal of SRs and MAs. Here, tools such as AMSTAR [18] come in handy to separate men of SRs from the boys.

A very common mistake is the mixing of apples with pears when it comes to collating studies on a topic. Usually, patient characteristics, disease status, inclusion criteria, kinds of interventions, and outcome assessments are diverse across primary studies included in SR/MA. This inevitably results in heterogeneity in their results. When a reader looks into the conclusions of a SR/MA, the patient characteristics of included studies should be systematically evaluated and compared with those they see in their clinics rather than jumping into interpreting the pooled results directly. It is a common mistake for physicians searching for results of a SR/MA to apply the meta-analytic conclusions in their practice without considering the possible differences between their patients and those enrolled in the included studies. Another important element to consider in the SR/MA is the quality of the primary studies included for the estimation of the treatment effect to be considered valid or trustworthy. Remember, an original study can be misleading, useless, or even harmful, even when it appears to be perfectly well designed, conducted, analyzed, and reported in a good journal. Several biases can affect the validity of the individual results, including selection bias, performance bias, detection bias, and attrition bias. So, if a meta-analysis has included potentially biased low-quality studies, then the conclusion of the meta-analysis will be likewise untrustworthy. For instance, an early MA published in Annals of Internal Medicine critically assessed the literature on the assessment of unprocessed red meat intake and risk for cardiometabolic outcomes concluded that there was low- to very-low-certainty evidence that higher red meat intake was associated with various health outcomes [67]. The methodology of the evidence of primary study was assessed to be not well performed.

Lastly, it is important to recognize that MA does not offer anything other than increase in statistical power; this feature can be an enemy, not a friend in some circumstances. It is well-known that publication bias exists. This means that SR/MA probably ends up including primary studies of small sample sizes published because they show statistical significance. Without a formal assessment of whether the sample of studies captured is representative or not, a SR/MA cannot really claim to present the "truth" in a manner that we believe does or we wish it would. Because when the results are pooled in MA, the overall sample size is increased and at the same time the probability of achieving statistical significance is also increased. The risk of type 2 error is reduced, but the risk of type 1 error may be increased. Thus, SR/MA may lead to an overoptimistic estimate of the results obtained. Suddenly, without due care and attention to detail, a powerful tool such as SR can readily become a source of misinformation and debate. This note of caution is best kept in mind whenever one reads a SR/MA.

2.7 Conclusion

With increasing focus on generating guidance and recommendations for shared decision-making while practicing evidence-based medicine, SRs are recognized as an essential tool to synthetize the available scientific research as well as to identify areas that are deficient in research. This chapter provided a brief step-by-step explanation of the conduct of an SR.

References

1. Khan KSKR, Antes G, Kleijnen J. Systematic reviews to support evidence-based medicine. London: Hodder Annold; 2011.
2. Khan KS, Kunz R, Kleijnen J, Antes G. Five steps to conducting a systematic review. J R Soc Med. 2003;96(3):118–21.
3. Khan KS, Bachmann LM, ter Riet G. Systematic reviews with individual patient data meta-analysis to evaluate diagnostic tests. Eur J Obstet Gynecol Reprod Biol. 2003;108(2):121–5.
4. Khan KS, Ball E, Fox CE, Meads C. Systematic reviews to evaluate causation: An overview of methods and application. Evid Based Med. 2012;17(5):137–41.
5. Nixon J, Khan KS, Kleijnen J. Summarising economic evaluations in systematic reviews: a new approach. BMJ. 2001;322(7302):1596–8.
6. Silva-Fernández L, Carmona L. Meta-analysis in the era of big data. Clin Rheumatol. 2019;38(8):2027–8.
7. Afnan MAM, Khan KS, Mol BW. Generating translatable evidence to improve patient care: the contribution of human factors. Reprod Biomed Online. 2020;41(3):353–6.
8. Fernández-Reino M English language use and profienciy of migrants in the UK-migration observatory: migration observatory; 2019. https://migrationobservatory.ox.ac.uk/resources/briefings/english-language-use-and-proficiency-of-migrants-in-the-uk/.
9. Gandhi TK, Burstin HR, Cook EF, Puopolo AL, Haas JS, Brennan TA, et al. Drug complications in outpatients. J Gen Intern Med. 2000;15(3):149–54.
10. Jih J, Vittinghoff E, Fernandez A. Patient-physician language concordance and use of preventive care services among limited English proficient Latinos and Asians. Public Health Rep. 2015;130(2):134–42.
11. Lehane D, Campion P. Interpreters: why should the NHS provide them? Br J Gen Pract. 2018;68(677):564–5.
12. Jaeger FN, Pellaud N, Laville B, Klauser P. Barriers to and solutions for addressing insufficient professional interpreter use in primary healthcare. BMC Health Serv Res. 2019;19:1.
13. Chien PF, Khan KS, Siassakos D. Registration of systematic reviews: PROSPERO. BJOG. 2012;119(8):903–5.
14. García-Martín M, Amezcua-Prieto C, Al Wattar B, Jørgensen JS, Bueno-Cavanillas A, Khan KS. Patient and public involvement in sexual and reproductive health: Time to properly integrate citizen's input into science. Int J Environ Res Public Health. 2020;17(21):1–12.
15. Cano-Ibáñez N, Zolfaghari Y, Amezcua-Prieto C, et al. Physician-Patient Language Discordance and Poor Health Outcomes: A Systematic Scoping Review. Frontiers in public health. 2021:9;629041. https://doi.org/10.3389/fpubh.2021.629041.
16. Eriksen MB, Frandsen TF. The impact of patient, intervention, comparison, outcome (Pico) as a search strategy tool on literature search quality: A systematic review. J Med Libr Assoc. 2018;106(4):420–31.
17. Stang A. Critical evaluation of the Newcastle-Ottawa scale for the assessment of the quality of nonrandomized studies in meta-analyses. Eur J Epidemiol. 2010;25(9):603–5.
18. Shea BJ, Grimshaw JM, Wells GA, Boers M, Andersson N, Hamel C, et al. Development of AMSTAR: A measurement tool to assess the methodological quality of systematic reviews. BMC Med Res Methodol. 2007;7:5.
19. Moher D, Liberati A, Tetzlaff J, Altman DG. Preferred reporting items for systematic reviews and meta-analyses: the PRISMA statement. BMJ. 2009;339:b2535.
20. Rogozinska E, Khan K. Grading evidence from test accuracy studies: What makes it challenging compared with the grading of effectiveness studies? Evid Based Med. 2017;22(3):81–4.
21. Khan KS, Borowiack E, Roos C, Kowalska M, Zapalska A, Mol BW, et al. Making GRADE accessible: a proposal for graphic display of evidence quality assessments. Evid Based Med. 2011;16(3):65–9.
22. Rogozińska E, Khan K. Grading evidence from test accuracy studies: what makes it challenging compared with the grading of effectiveness studies? Evid Based Med. 2017;22(3):81–4.

23. Nothnagel K. RBT: vote counting and meta-analysis. In: Empirical research within resource-based theory: a meta-analysis of the central propositions. Wiesbaden: Gabler; 2008. p. 143–99.
24. Wandersman A, Alia KA, Cook B, Ramaswamy R. Integrating empowerment evaluation and quality improvement to achieve healthcare improvement outcomes. BMJ Qual Saf. 2015;24(10):645–52.
25. Auerbach AD, Landefeld CS, Shojania KG. The tension between needing to improve care and knowing how to do it. N Engl J Med. 2007;357(6):608–13.
26. Marshall M, Pronovost P, Dixon-Woods M. Promotion of improvement as a science. Lancet. 2013;381(9864):419–21.
27. (IOM) IoM. Clinical practice guidelines we can trust; 2011.
28. Johnston A, Kelly SE, Hsieh SC, Skidmore B, Wells GA. Systematic reviews of clinical practice guidelines: a methodological guide. J Clin Epidemiol. 2019;108:64–76.
29. Khan KS, Borowiack E, Roos C, Kowalska M, Zapalska A, Mol BW, et al. Making GRADE accessible: a proposal for graphic display of evidence quality assessments. Evid Based Med. 2011;16(3):65–9.
30. Rogozinska E, Khan K. Grading evidence from test accuracy studies: what makes it challenging compared with the grading of effectiveness studies? Evid Based Med. 2017;22(3):81–4.
31. Kulier R, Gee H, Khan KS. Five steps from evidence to effect: exercising clinical freedom to implement research findings. BJOG. 2008;115(10):1197–202.
32. Vernooij RW, Sanabria AJ, Sola I, Alonso-Coello P, Martinez GL. Guidance for updating clinical practice guidelines: a systematic review of methodological handbooks. Implement Sci. 2014;9:3.
33. Maes-Carballo M, Munoz-Nunez I, Martin-Diaz M, Mignini L, Bueno-Cavanillas A, Khan KS. Shared decision making in breast cancer treatment guidelines: development of a quality assessment tool and a systematic review. Health Expect. 2020;23:1045.
34. Maes-Carballo M, Mignini L, Martin-Diaz M, Bueno-Cavanillas A, Khan KS. Quality and reporting of clinical guidelines for breast cancer treatment: a systematic review. Breast. 2020;53:201–11.
35. Amezcua-Prieto C, Fernandez-Luna JM, Huete-Guadix JF, Bueno-Cavanillas A, Khan KS. Artificial intelligence and automation of systematic reviews in women's health. Curr Opin Obstet Gynecol. 2020;32(5):335–41.
36. Elwyn G, Frosch D, Thomson R, Joseph-Williams N, Lloyd A, Kinnersley P, et al. Shared decision making: a model for clinical practice. J Gen Intern Med. 2012;27(10):1361–7.
37. Levit LA, Nass S, Ganz P. Delivering high-quality cancer care: charting a new course for a system in crisis. Washington: The National Academies Press; 2013.
38. Schoenfeld EM, Mader S, Houghton C, Wenger R, Probst MA, Schoenfeld DA, et al. The effect of shared decision making on patients' likelihood of filing a complaint or lawsuit: a simulation study. Ann Emerg Med. 2019;74(1):126–36.
39. Estado BOd. Ley 41/2002 básica reguladora de la autonomía del paciente y de derechos y obligaciones en materia de información y documentación clínica. [Basic Law 41/2002 regulating the autonomy of the patient and rights and obligations regarding information and clinical documentation], BOE; 2002.
40. Senate and House of Representatives. Patient Protection and Affordable Care Act. HR 3590. Washington; 2010.
41. Department of Health. Equity and excellence: liberating the NHS. London; 2010.
42. International Shared Decision Making Society; 2018.
43. AECC. Estudio de investigación "Necesidades no clínicas de los pacientes con cáncer y sus acompañantes en España: una visión multidisciplinar". La mitad de los pacientes oncológicos no participa en la toma de decisiones sobre su tratamiento. [Research study "Non-clinical needs of cancer patients and their companions in Spain: a multidisciplinary vision" . Half of cancer patients do not participate in decision-making about their treatment]. 2018.
44. The Patients Association, UK; 2018.
45. Legare F, Thompson-Leduc P. Twelve myths about shared decision making. Patient Educ Couns. 2014;96(3):281–6.

46. Savelberg W, Boersma LJ, Smidt M, Goossens MFJ, Hermanns R, van der Weijden T. Does lack of deeper understanding of shared decision making explains the suboptimal performance on crucial parts of it? An example from breast cancer care. Eur J Oncol Nurs. 2019;38:92–7.
47. Stacey D, Hill S, McCaffery K, Boland L, Lewis KB, Horvat L. Shared decision making interventions: theoretical and empirical evidence with implications for health literacy. Stud Health Technol Inform. 2017;240:263–83.
48. Gillick MR. Re-engineering shared decision-making. J Med Ethics. 2015;41(9):785–8.
49. Volk RJ, Llewellyn-Thomas H, Stacey D, Elwyn G. Ten years of the International Patient Decision Aid Standards Collaboration: evolution of the core dimensions for assessing the quality of patient decision aids. BMC Med Inform Decis Mak. 2013;13:1.
50. Staveley I, Sullivan P. We need more guidance on shared decision making. Br J Gen Pract. 2015;65(641):663–4.
51. Légaré FAR, Stacey D, Turcotte S, Kryworuchkolan J, Lyddiatt GA, Politi MC, Thomson R, Elwyn G, Donner-Banzhoff N. Interventions for increasing the use of shared decision making by healthcare professionals. Cochrane Database Syst Rev. 2018;7(7):CD006732.
52. Elwyn G, Frosch DL, Kobrin S. Implementing shared decision-making: consider all the consequences. Implement Sci. 2016;11:114.
53. Agoritsas T, Heen AF, Brandt L, Alonso-Coello P, Kristiansen A, Akl EA, et al. Decision aids that really promote shared decision making: the pace quickens. BMJ. 2015;350:g7624.
54. Elwyn G, Lloyd A, Joseph-Williams N, Cording E, Thomson R, Durand MA, et al. Option Grids: shared decision making made easier. Patient Educ Couns. 2013;90(2):207–12.
55. Holmes-Rovner M, Valade D, Orlowski C, Draus C, Nabozny-Valerio B, Keiser S. Implementing shared decision-making in routine practice: barriers and opportunities. Health Expect. 2000;3(3):182–91.
56. Wieringa TH, Rodriguez-Gutierrez R, Spencer-Bonilla G, de Wit M, Ponce OJ, Sanchez-Herrera MF, et al. Decision aids that facilitate elements of shared decision making in chronic illnesses: a systematic review. Syst Rev. 2019;8(1):121.
57. Bomhof-Roordink H, Gartner FR, Stiggelbout AM, Pieterse AH. Key components of shared decision making models: a systematic review. BMJ Open. 2019;9(12):e031763.
58. Hussain JA, Flemming K, Murtagh FE, Johnson MJ. Patient and health care professional decision-making to commence and withdraw from renal dialysis: a systematic review of qualitative research. Clin J Am Soc Nephrol. 2015;10(7):1201–15.
59. Williams N, Fleming C, Doubleday A. Patient and provider perspectives on shared decision making: a systematic review of the peer-reviewed literature. J Comp Eff Res. 2017;6(8):683–92.
60. Pollard S, Bansback N, Bryan S. Physician attitudes toward shared decision making: a systematic review. Patient Educ Couns. 2015;98(9):1046–57.
61. Wyatt KD, List B, Brinkman WB, Prutsky Lopez G, Asi N, Erwin P, et al. Shared decision making in pediatrics: a systematic review and meta-analysis. Acad Pediatr. 2015;15(6):573–83.
62. Saheb Kashaf M, McGill ET, Berger ZD. Shared decision-making and outcomes in type 2 diabetes: a systematic review and meta-analysis. Patient Educ Couns. 2017;100(12):2159–71.
63. Muller E, Strukava A, Scholl I, Harter M, Diouf NT, Legare F, et al. Strategies to evaluate healthcare provider trainings in shared decision-making (SDM): a systematic review of evaluation studies. BMJ Open. 2019;9(6):e026488.
64. Shay LA, Lafata JE. Where is the evidence? A systematic review of shared decision making and patient outcomes. Med Decis Making. 2015;35(1):114–31.
65. WHO. Coronavirus disease (COVID-19). Geneva: WHO; 2020.
66. Balla M, Merugu GP, Patel M, Koduri NM, Gayam V, Adapa S, et al. COVID-19, modern pandemic: a systematic review from front-line health care providers' perspective. J Clin Med Res. 2020;12(4):215–29.
67. Zeraatkar D, Han MA, Guyatt GH, Vernooij RWM, El Dib R, Cheung K, et al. Red and processed meat consumption and risk for all-cause mortality and cardiometabolic outcomes a systematic review and meta-analysis of cohort studies. Ann Intern Med. 2019;171(10):703–10.

Chapter 3
Personal Branding and Social Customer Relationship Management in Science, Nurturing Research?

Ricardo Cunha Lopes

3.1 Introduction

When we think about brands, we associate it with a specific product or corporation's unique attribute for marketing effects. Until recently, the theory of branding was limited to the consumer-product relationship. But, with the amplification of the personal development phenomenon, branding steps into this area, leading to specific personal activities and named personal branding. Despite the current hype, this phenomenon is not new and has a long history. Brands are not a modern invention. Like Elvis Presley, the Pharaoh was also a brand—his image meant much more to millions of admirers than the Pharaoh himself, and after his death, they continued to "follow" him for a long time [1]. The essential elements of a person as a brand are the importance of standing out, presenting an authentic and distinct message.

Also, successful brands harness the community's power to increase their awareness, develop engagement, improve outcomes, and build brand loyalty. Community relationship marketing relies on the principles of relationship marketing theory. Relationship marketing hinges on the development of lasting customer-brand bonds, which creates a sustainable competitive advantage [2]. Social media platforms create social and structural bonds with the community through the co-creation process, promoting engagement [3].

The level of expertise in the research community has evolved considerably. The pressure on university scientists to present their work in high quantity is relentless. More exposure means more prestige for a researcher's department—and the prestige will translate into more support from the university. Consequently, it has become increasingly necessary for scientists to cultivate a personal brand and

R. C. Lopes (✉)
FEUP - Faculty of Engineering, University of Porto, Porto, Portugal

G. C. Di Renzo (ed.), *Essential Writing, Communication and Narrative Skills for Medical Scientists Before and After the COVID Era*,
https://doi.org/10.1007/978-3-030-84954-2_3

expand their network connections, developing their own social community relationship management.

We highlight two motivations for which personal branding give an edge for a researcher, especially a young researcher.

- *Brands Move With You*
- Scientists are no longer associated with a single university or research field for their entire careers. There are several reasons for this: (1) the need to change institutions to advance in a career, (2) shifts in scientific agenda, and (3) unstable funding. For these reasons, personal branding can facilitate dynamic career development
- *Your Own Network is Your Most Important Tool*
- The explosion of scientific publications that overwhelm the publication system has made it impossible the traditional peer review protocol to work or for the scientific community to evaluate on-time scientific research. Due to an overabundance of articles awaiting reviews or publication, decisions like suspending all new publishing submissions sign that future researchers need to develop a second tier of communication with peers, to stand out.

3.2 Developing Your Brand

3.2.1 The Personal Brand

A brand is a relationship. It is not a contrived image, or snappy statement, or an artificial veneer. A branded relationship is a single type of connection that involves trust and only happens when two individuals believe that there is a direct link between their value systems. Attachments matter.

Everybody already has a brand. Your brand reflects who you are and is expressed by what you do and how you do it. Developing a personal brand that is clear, complete, and valuable to others, you are building a perception in others' minds. A perception you can nurture and control. The core objective of personal branding is to market oneself to society [4]. This marketing-driven trend is described as a group of features that distinguish one individual from another. Establishing a unique personal identity and developing an active communication approach of one's brand identity to a specific target market and evaluating its impact on one's image and reputation [5–7]. In other words, personal branders manage extended self online and offline [8].

Self-branding entails that individuals think of themselves as products to be marketed to a broad audience in the hopes of becoming more economically competitive. The discourse of self-branding directs self-presentation in a very specific, instrumental way, requiring constant self-reflection and evaluation in constructing a "strong brand".

Self-branding entails that individuals think of themselves as products to be marketed to a broad audience in the hopes of becoming more economically competitive. The discourse of self-branding directs self-presentation in a very specific, instrumental way, requiring constant self-reflection and evaluation in constructing a "strong brand".

This self-branding approach entails that individuals think of themselves as products to be marketed to a broad audience, to become more relevant and economically competitive. Self-branding" discourse directs self-presentation in a precise, instrumental way, requiring constant self-reflection and evaluation in constructing a strong brand, consistent throughout all interactions [9, 10]. It is based on an individual's personal or professional reputation, resulting in personal or organization revenue from a career management perspective if maintained and sustained according to the market needs [11].

The Human Brand Theory [12] provides a conceptual lens for this approach. It proposes the paths in which a digital mediated persona can evolve into a personal brand.

A Human Brand offers a feeling of attachment to his/her audience and yields positive marketing results by fulfilling needs. The Human Brand Theory identifies three vertices. First, media personas such as celebrities, athletes, and politicians can be considered human brands if they meet a set of conditions such as a unique personality or ability, thereby becoming the subject of marketing communications efforts. An individual's brand reflects his or her skills, abilities, and lifestyle [13, 14].

Second, the theory identifies three psychological needs that create strong relationships with their followers. Following the acronym ARC, they are:

- Autonomy: a feeling of self-determination in choice and action.
- Relatedness: a sense of intimacy.
- Competence: a feeling of proficiency.
- It concludes that, if a human brand fulfills these needs, these individuals will develop a strong emotional bond with the human brand.

Third, the theory proposes that this strong relationship leads human brands to create successful marketing effects. Consumers loyal to a brand have a higher probability of embracing that brand's product extension by showing an automatic transfer of positive effects from the brand to another branded product [15]. The same holds in the human brand context. The attachment formed to a human brand facilitates the effective transfer of positive feelings from that human brand to the products/brands that human brand endorses. This effect is referred to as attachment transfer [12].

Before the advent of digital media, successful personal brands operated in an offline world that used tactics such as speaking conferences, meet and greets, white papers, etc. But the time has changed, and those channels, on their own, are no longer enough. Today, digital personal branding, which includes such methods as podcasts, blogs, and online social media, must be a part of the personal brand-development mix. The most effective and successful practitioners will find the right balance between offline and online personal branding. The practice of personal branding relies on a combination of offline and online presentation of the self. It is an ongoing process that requires constant interactions with others online and offline [13].

During the past decade, online personal branding has evolved, which can be attributed to the proliferation of computer-mediated communication and the evolution of social media that have enabled people to use the internet to create and foster their identity [16]. Social media acts like an information exchange system whereby identity is created and consumed by online audiences. These systems enable individuals to build their persona, creating and presenting a distinct representation of themselves. Therefore, an individual can be selective in their self-presentation techniques [17]. Social media marketing has fundamentally changed the traditional brand/business-development model. From the traditional model, where the mantra it's not what you know, but who you know, social media changed that mantra to a model that believes it's not who you know, but who knows you. The shift continues to evolve through new online tools and platforms that individuals use to share information, such as blogs, social networking sites, wikis, podcasts, and shared media, building new digital communities.

3.2.2 The Movement Toward Digital

In the last decade, community relationships evolved to a more sophisticated level due to an ever-evolving challenging environment with new social routines and new technologies brought by Web 2.0. The collaborative web 2.0 is highlighted with platforms like wikis, blogs, and social media networks that foster relationships, collaboration, and sharing among. The social network concept is defined as a system that contains nodes such as people, groups, and other organizations connected by edges that link them together by a range of relationships [18]. Web 2.0 is also known as social media, and it represents a revolution in how people communicate. It can be described as online media networks that use internet-based applications to connect, share, and promote user-generated content, to enable peer-to-peer relationships and real-time interaction [19, 20].

The sheer diversity and number of opportunities to publicize oneself have changed the way individuals, consumers and businesses interact with each other [21]. Online personal branding is taking shape through conventional e-marketing tools such as personal blogs and e-mail and web 2.0 platforms like YouTube, Twitter, Facebook, and LinkedIn, which are transforming the way the internet and self-branding are approached [7, 21, 22]. A personal brand is built on a combination of who you know, what you know, how you share knowledge, and how quickly you bring your point of view to the audience. In the past, individuals and organizations used to control communication activities and personal brand-building by pushing information out. Today, "push" is giving way to "dialogue," where peer to peer-driven information is becoming a meaningful way to invite prospects into relationships that can be transformed into new opportunities.

The most significant impact of web 2.0 platforms on personal branding is that it has simplified the process and shortened the time to build brand awareness. In the offline world, only leading researchers have a stage to deliver their message, but today, everyone can broadcast their findings and thoughts via a social media platform. Nevertheless, online should not be a replacement for offline, personal branding. People buy from people, and face-to-face relationship building is, still, the baseline of any personal branding strategy.

Personal branding demands content, frequency, and consistency of interaction. A researcher can longer count on the goodwill built by speaking or writing once a year to enhance their brand and need to commit to using tools like blogs and social media platforms regularly to gain social capital. The downside effect is that this global publication rush accelerates irrelevancy. Effective personal brand development requires dedication and commitment to communication through timely postings, comments to peers, and updates to whatever social media platform the researcher employs. Frequency of communication equates directly to relevancy, and relevancy is the basis for creating the perception of thought leadership. Publications in group forums and social media platforms provide a first-to-thought awareness that digitally literate researchers need to deploy in their branding tactics.

Establishing the right balance between offline and online actions is a common challenge. Different generations of researchers don't approach the challenge in the same way. Younger researchers need to recognize face-to-face relationships and research-development activities, and senior researchers need to incorporate digital personal branding into their career development habits. The movement toward a digital personal brand should trigger a shift of personal marketing time and resources, not an addition. Consequently, it may be time to create or adjust your brand plan, as this will be the roadmap that determines the right balance between offline and online personal branding activities.

3.2.3 Personal Branding Framework

Most individuals already have a personal brand regardless of their consciousness. Individuals possess intrinsic personal branding due to personality qualities, experience and development, and communication with others whether they know it or not [23].

Three key components must guide the development of the framework to ensure your strong personal brand's development:

- Distinctive: You stand for something. You have a point of view.
- Relevant: What you stand for connects to what someone else considers to be important.

- Consistent: People come to believe in a relationship based on the consistency of behaviors they experience or observe from you.

There are many different formats for developing a personal marketing plan. Taking into consideration the needed balance between offline and online, we propose the following framework.

#1. Make your statement	A power statement A concise way of letting peers, followers, and referral sources know what you do and how and why your research is different. It must be short, accurate, and immediately understandable
#2. Design the strategy	Conduct a situational and SWOT analysis Identify opportunities (peers, themes, events, publishers) and your target audience Define your unique research proposition and differentiation Start the process of determining how you are going to promote the brand Online, reserve a domain name and a name on leading social networks Identify the online communities you should join and the online communities that you might wish to build and own Design a publication plan that aims to engage with the community
# 3. Define the goals	Establish measurable goals Offline, goals might include number of articles written, presentations given, etc. Online, database entries, webinar invitations, social referrals, SEO rankings or followers are rule of thumb
#4. Curate your brand	Offline, step into community and association involvement Cultivate relationships with journalists in traditional print media Make grand rounds presentations, university lectures, TED talks, and presentations at national meetings Online, secure a clear footprint Develop profiles on social networks such as LinkedIn, Facebook, twitter, and ResearchGate Publish own content and share the most relevant from third party Improve your position in Google Make sure your profile on your research center or university web site is current, accurate, and strategically linked within and outside of the site Contribute to your research center or university digital media communications (e.g., newsletters, podcasts, webinars) that are also linked to your social media profile(s) Showcase your personal brand, reaching out to others in your niche and dialoguing on publications in your area of expertise with useful insights

3.3 Closing Remarks

Personal branding is the beginning of a fantastic journey that aims to develop a new communication layer for researchers. The edited self results from transparency, audience, intimacy, and authenticity, motivating social media users to construct consistent online profiles carefully [24]. The curated personal brand caters to the professional (research-related) future audience.

The curated self extends from online to offline. Curation is used to construct, build, and perform individualized identities across networks that bridge online and offline experiences.

While personal branding is articulated as relevant for young researchers entering a research career, personal branding has also become necessary for senior researchers and throughout the Academia hierarchy.

Finally, as noted earlier, building a strong personal brand takes courage—because consistency takes courage. The way to make a distinctive, enduring, positive impression on someone else is to ensure that who you are, what you say you are, and what that person experiences from you are the same, time and time again.

References

1. Harari YN. Homo Deus: a brief history of tomorrow. Barcelona: Debate; 2016.
2. Bowden J. Customer engagement: a framework for assessing customer-brand relationships: the case of the restaurant industry. J Hosp Market Manag. 2009;18(6):574–96.
3. Strauss J, Frost R. E-marketing. 2001;
4. Johnson KM. The importance of personal branding in social media: educating students to create and manage their personal brand. Int J Educ Soc Sci. 2017;4(1):7.
5. Brooks AK, Anumudu C. Identity development in personal branding instruction: social narratives and online Brand Management in a global economy. Adult Learn. 2016;27(1):23–9. https://doi.org/10.1177/1045159515616968.
6. Wetsch LR. A personal branding assignment using social media. J Advert Educ. 2012;16(1):30–6. https://doi.org/10.1177/109804821201600106.
7. Kleppinger CA, Cain J. Personal digital branding as a professional asset in the digital age. Am J Pharm Educ. 2015;79(6):79. https://doi.org/10.5688/ajpe79679.
8. Belk RW. Extended self in a digital world: table 1. J Consum Res. 2013;40(3):477–500. https://doi.org/10.1086/671052.
9. Wee L, Brooks A. Personal branding and the commodification of reflexivity. Cult Soc. 2010;4(1):45–62. https://doi.org/10.1177/1749975509356754.
10. Whitmer JM. You are your brand: Self-branding and the marketization of self. Sociol Compass. 2019;13(3):e12662. https://doi.org/10.1111/soc4.12662.
11. Mohammed E, Steyn R. Personal branding: a systematic review of the research and design strategies used reported in journal articles relating to critical elements of personal branding. In: Proceedings of the international conference on business and management dynamics 2016: Sustainable economies in the information economy. AOSIS; 2016. pp. 1–9. http://www.icbmd.org/index.php/ICBMD/2016/paper/view/71
12. Thomson M. Human brands: investigating antecedents to consumers' strong attachments to celebrities. J Mark. 2006;70(3):104–19. https://doi.org/10.1509/jmkg.70.3.104.
13. Hearn A. `Meat, mask, burden`. J Consum Cult. 2008;8(2):197–217. https://doi.org/10.1177/1469540508090086.
14. Moulard JG, Garrity CP, Rice DH. What makes a human brand authentic? Identifying the antecedents of celebrity authenticity. Psychol Mark. 2015;32(2):173–86. https://doi.org/10.1002/mar.20771.
15. Yeung CWM, Wyer RS. Does loving a brand mean loving its products? The role of brand-elicited affect in brand extension evaluations. J Market Res. 2005;42(4):495–506. https://doi.org/10.1509/jmkr.2005.42.4.495.
16. Albright JM, Simmens E. Flirting, cheating, dating, and mating in a virtual world. Oxford: Oxford University Press; 2014.

17. Rosenberg J, Egbert N. Online impression management: personality traits and concerns for secondary goals as predictors of self-presentation tactics on Facebook. J Comput Commun. 2011;17(1):1–18. https://doi.org/10.1111/j.1083-6101.2011.01560.x.
18. Anshari M, Almunawar MN, Lim SA, Al-Mudimigh A. Customer relationship management and big data enabled: personalization & customization of services. Appl Comput Informatics. 2019;15(2):94–101. https://doi.org/10.1016/j.aci.2018.05.004.
19. Dwivedi YK, Kapoor KK, Chen H. Social media marketing and advertising. Mark Rev. 2015;15(3):289–309.
20. Evans D, McKee J, Bratton S. Social media marketing: the next generation of business engagement. London: Wiley; 2010.
21. Taiminen H, Karjaluoto H. The usage of digital marketing channels in SMEs. J Small Bus Enterp Dev. 2015;22:633–51.
22. Gandini A. Digital work: self-branding and social capital in the freelance knowledge economy. Mark Theory. 2016;16(1):123–41. https://doi.org/10.1177/1470593115607942.
23. Rangarajan D, Gelb BD, Vandaveer A. Strategic personal branding—and how it pays off. Bus Horiz. 2017;60(5):657–66.
24. Marwick AE, Boyd D. I tweet honestly, I tweet passionately: twitter users, context collapse, and the imagined audience. New Media Soc. 2011;13(1):114–33. https://doi.org/10.1177/1461444810365313.

Chapter 4
Essentials on Writing a Paper for a Peer Reviewed Journal

Marta Maes-Carballo, Khalid Saeed Khan, and Naomi Cano-Ibáñez

4.1 Introduction

Writing a medical article that will be accepted for publication by journal editors and peer-reviewers is not an easy task. Most doctors find it difficult to express their studies, which have taken much time and effort to research, in a manner that convinces referees of medical journals. It is necessary to know that writing an article is not creative writing but a piece of science for which the process and structure are extremely formulaic. Vital requirements for achieving the publication of an article include many things besides the choice of an important topic and the conduct of good research itself. What matters is whether journal editors consider it worth reporting. Authors need to rigidly follow an accepted medical journal article structure and use a suitable scientific language. Being successful in a publication requires

M. Maes-Carballo
Department of Preventive Medicine and Public Health, University of Granada, Granada, Spain

Department of General Surgery, Complexo Hospitalario de Ourense, Ourense, Spain

K. S. Khan
Department of Preventive Medicine and Public Health, University of Granada, Granada, Spain

CIBER of Epidemiology and Public Health (CIBERESP), Madrid, Spain

N. Cano-Ibáñez (✉)
Department of Preventive Medicine and Public Health, University of Granada, Granada, Spain

CIBER of Epidemiology and Public Health (CIBERESP), Madrid, Spain

Instituto de Investigación Biosanitaria de Granada (ibs. GRANADA), Granada, Spain
e-mail: ncaiba@ugr.es

G. C. Di Renzo (ed.), *Essential Writing, Communication and Narrative Skills for Medical Scientists Before and After the COVID Era*,
https://doi.org/10.1007/978-3-030-84954-2_4

authors to make a good impression on editors because without their approval they cannot give what clinician readers want from them. Furthermore, dealing with peer review could be challenging, and there is not enough good guidance on it. Procrastination limits the opportunities for revision of the draft manuscript to a higher standard ahead of the submission deadline. Knowing the journal's paper assessment and publishing process should be a must. Every author should try writing an article in the best way possible because a paper rejected once will probably also be rejected on resubmission.

The aim of this chapter is to familiarize new authors with unwritten rules that will help in the publication of their manuscripts, giving writing tips to increase the probability of a manuscript being accepted on first submission.

4.2 Manuscript Assessment and Publishing Process

Understanding the manuscript assessment and publishing process is important in order to have chances to be successful. Figure 4.1 shows the major steps involved in publishing a research paper. The first step should be identifying an important

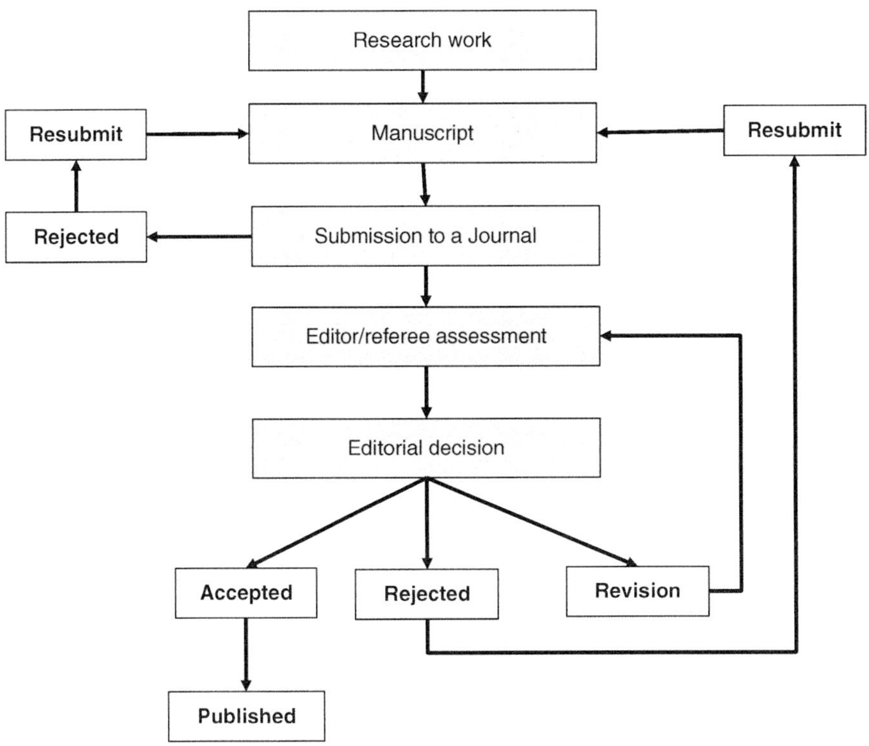

Fig. 4.1 Flow-diagram of publication process

research question which should be of value to practice as well as being interesting to share. Once the research work is completed, the second step should be the identification of a relevant journal and studying its aims and instructions; writing the manuscript should directly adhere to the rules of the journal. The third step should be the submission of the manuscript with all relevant supporting materials and checklists. In the fourth step, the manuscript will enter a multi-stage assessment process. This step will only progress if the manuscript is well-formatted and is suitable according to the aims and scope of the journal. Initially, the manuscript will be subjected to basic administrative assessments (including plagiarism check and compliance with journal style) and then read by an editor to assess quality and relevance; a proportion of articles will be rejected at this initial stage. The second stage will be peer-reviewed. Finally, a decision will be taken: rejected or revision required (revision of the paper will be needed per comment followed by resubmission, but that alone will not guarantee acceptance; quality of the response will matter). Acceptance without any revisions is rare. Rejection is common. The acceptance rate across journals vary, being 5–30% depending on journal ranking and manuscript type among other factors.

4.3 Focus on Key Elements of the Research Question

It is necessary to start with a structured research question [1] that will help to focus the paper in a way that appears a coherent whole to the editors. In the past many writing teachers have recommended to start jotting down all the ideas on a black piece of paper. In the modern day, this approach can be easily replicated on the computer, tablet, or mobile phone. Table 4.1 represents an example of the structured research question for a study already published [2].

After this initial work has been done, the ideas must be located into sections described in the mnemonic IMRAD: Introduction, Methods, Results, and Discussion (Table 4.2). Unfortunately this does not cover two key elements, Title and Abstract, sections that are the key to success in publications. No work nowadays is done by individual researchers. Teamwork is what gets us there. The writing plans should be discussed with the team, with whom the writing tasks can be distributed. This allows addition of new perspectives that may increase the chances of success in publishing [3]. Beware though that the old adage "too many cooks spoil the broth" also applies in scientific writing.

Table 4.1 The focal points of a manuscript with an example [2]

Participants: Women with breast cancer
Intervention: Clinical practice guidelines (CPGs) and consensus statements (CSs) for shared decision-making with participants
Comparison: CPGs and CSs without advice on shared decision-making
Outcome: General quality of CPGs and CSs concerning shared decision-making
Design and methods: Systematic review of literature

Table 4.2 Title, abstract, and IMRAD structure of an article

Title
Abstract
Introduction
1. Brief background (disease prevalence, burden on) 2. Justification for the current study based on gaps in previous works 3. Objectives of the study
Material and methods
(Follow related guidelines for reporting) 1. Approvals and registrations 2. Definitions of the study participants, interventions/exposures, and outcomes 3. Design of the research and methods to reduce bias 4. Statistical methods 5. Patient and public involvement
Results
1. Description of baseline characteristics 2. Description of the results 3. Figures and tables
Discussion
1. Summary of major findings 2. Strengths and limitations of the study 3. Comparison with findings of other studies 4. Implication of the results for practice 5. Lessons for future research

4.4 Title, Abstract, and Introduction

It is an essential part of the manuscript as the initial assessment by editor (Fig. 4.1) typically analyzes the Title, the Abstract, and the Introduction. It is these that make the first impression. To avoid rejection at the first assessment requires authors to focus on the proper devotion of attention to detail in writing and rewriting these sections. The greater the number of times these are revised, the higher the chance that they are free of errors and convincing. Writing abstract on the last day before submission is a classical recipe for rejection. If the editors find any problems in the Title, Abstract, or Introduction, they will probably reject the paper without reading the rest of the text and without peer-review.

It is a common myth that title, abstract, and introduction should be written at the end of the writing process, just before submission. The first opportunity to write the abstract should be taken at the time of writing the protocol, the second at the time of registering the study, and the third at the time of initiating the manuscript writing process with results known. The process of writing title, abstract, and introduction should not be delayed. According to the type of article, there are different checklists that help with the process of writing (e.g., CONSORT [4, 5], PRISMA [6, 7] or STROBE [8] checklists) in addition to the instructions of the journal.

Title and subtitle: The Title should be short and self-explanatory for it to be attractive to editors and peer-reviewers. It should induce them to read the rest of the paper and help them see how it can create an impact when published. Furthermore, it is a vital requirement for a good search engine optimization, which permits for the article to be found in the worldwide web and in different databases. Some of the four key elements shown in Table 4.1 should appear in the title and subtitle: participants, intervention or exposure and outcomes (title), and study design (subtitle). Too much information can be counterproductive and messy. The subtitle is usually required by reporting guidelines to state the study design, and you can also give some salient features of the methods or statistics for added importance. To be suc cinct, the title and subtitle together should be no longer than the length of a tweet. It should preferably not include question marks and abbreviations. Finally, the title has always to comply with the journal instructions in addition to adhering to reporting guidelines.

4.5 Abstract

The Abstract can be considered as a miniature version of the article, and it should offer a brief summary of each of the main sections of the article. This section is the most important part of the manuscript to focus on. The Abstract is where authors come forward giving a good first impression. Only if the abstract is well written and contains the main information about the scientific work done, the editors will continue reading the article further. The abstract can be presented in two main types: unstructured and structured. In the unstructured abstract, there are no divisions of the text and the information is presented in a paragraph or narrative form. The structured abstract is composed of several short paragraphs that describe the most relevant of each of the parts of the manuscript.

Depending on the guidelines of each journal, the abstract may be of one type or another. Even if structured abstract is not required, it can be deployed to draft text. Once drafted, the headings removed to combine the text into the unstructured format required. According to structured abstract, and taking into consideration that this structure can vary between journals, the most common headings include: background, objective(s), methods (design), results, and conclusions. It should be able to stand alone, avoid undefined abbreviations or references to the main text, and follow the instructions of the journal and those of the reporting guidelines. The abstract is succinct because it is limited to 200–300 words by most journals. The conclusions of the abstract should be based on the main results of the study presented in the paper, not based on the findings of the previous studies. Nowadays, the possibility of setting a Video abstract, a 60 to 90 seconds short video presenting your work, is sometimes available depending on the journal.

Introduction: The Introduction of a scientific paper informs of the purpose and importance of the work that will be presented. This section should be written after Title and Abstract, and, like the entire manuscript, the author must plan, select, and order its content in a logical sequence of ideas. It should be usually a brief section of about 250 to 600 words. It must first include a paragraph about the temporal and spatial contextualization of the study topic, that is, describe the disease burden in terms of prevalence, life quality impact, health economic costs, etc. Then there should be a paragraph about what is known and what is not known about the scientific question, a section that gives and overview of the weaknesses of previous studies to justify the need for the study being presented. And, lastly the objective(s) of the study should be presented, replicating the same hypothesis written in the Abstract. Introduction is one the most difficult sections to write due to the need to be brief while remaining relevant and innovative. The introductory paragraphs set the tone and quality of the manuscript.

As we mentioned previously, the Introduction should establish the necessity of the subject matter of the work but it does not take up too much space to develop it. So, the general concept using three paragraphs outlined above (Table 4.3) should be strictly applied. The first paragraph should be a brief background (participants, interventions, outcomes, and disease burden) that could be backed by current references identified using a systematic review search filter in databases [9]. This is not a place for text book knowledge. It should be concise, explanatory, and instructive. Scientific references related to the topic should support all the text in this section. The second paragraph should explain why the study was undertaken by giving reasons to justify the need for addressing the specific issue. The weaknesses of previous researches should be politely highlighted in order to explain the knowledge gap that exists which the study will address. The third and last paragraph should explain the objective, including the design of the study and focusing on what we could expect to answer from reading the manuscript.

4.6 Tables and Figures

The evidence of the article could be contained in the figures and the tables. They are the most important key part of the results and their footnotes should be well-explained. If a reader moves from Abstract directly to figures and tables, they should find everything they need right there, without the need to go into the Methods and Results sections. For this reason, it is requirement that figures and tables should be stand-alone and must be fully self-explanatory without the need to refer to the text. Moreover, they should be simple and including numerical data. Thus, tables and figures complement the text and help to a quick and accurate understanding of the results. The main objective of tables and figures is to emphasize the most significant

Table 4.3 Parts and explanation of the introduction

Parts of the introduction	Explanation
1. Brief background	The current situation of the main topic should be given
2. Importance of the current study and gaps in previous works	Why was the study undertaken? Weakness of previous studies should be highlighted to justify our study
3. Main purpose of the study	The objective of the study

data and summarize the main results. Information can be presented in many manners, horizontal or vertical. Three-dimensional graphs or solitary pie charts are confusing and should not be used. All data symbols and abbreviations should be defined. Figures and tables could be used for explaining methods and results in an easier way, and references should appear within the text. Data should be synthesized in the correct order, excluding trivial values and eradicating unnecessary words. Legends should be short and complementary to the text. The advantages of using figures and tables have been demonstrated in that they increase efficiency saving time required for understanding. The accuracy of the interpretation, when presented in a figure, is greater than in a table, and it takes longer to read a table than a figure. Depending on the format of the scientific journal, the tables are placed at the end of the manuscript or in separate files at the time of submission. They are incorporated in the text at the time of typesetting and formatting following acceptance.

4.7 Methods

This section should be meticulously explained by providing enough detail and references in line with specific reporting guidelines. It is usually divided into various sections: ethics approval and registration [10], design of the study, participants, interventions and outcomes, data collection procedures, statistical analyses, and patient and public involvement. Accuracy and clarity must be the goals due to the fact Methods give validity to the findings. The main aim of this section is to permit other researchers to evaluate if the study is well-designed and appropriate for the study objective. The literature references should be used as pillars to construct this section. Statistical analysis should be done to accept or reject the hypothesis presented in the Introduction. It should essentially contain well-written language because switching the point of view between passive and active voice misleads and distracts the reader. Some studies have stated that Materials and Methods is the only part of a manuscript in which passive voice predominantly overrides the use of the active voice [11–14].

4.8 Results

The Results section, in line with reporting guidelines, should have at least two important parts: the presentation of data and output of the data analysis both supported by Tables and Figures. The Results must be written in an explicit and unambiguous way using precise numerical data to support the statement. Only relevant results related to the purpose of the study should be specified. They should be presented in a proper order, following the order of the objective(s) of the study. Insignificant results should not be omitted as negative findings are important. When giving the effects and associations observed, the Results must report numerical data and statistical terms, i.e., confidence intervals, level of significance, etc. using the statistical evaluation specified in the Methods section.

4.9 Discussion and Conclusion

The aim of the Discussion section is to state the principal findings, their validity, and their implications. The strength and weaknesses of the study (risk of bias) should be reviewed. The limitations regarding comparison with other studies should be given. Unanswered questions and future research should be taken into account too. Table 4.4 resumes one suggested structure for discussion of scientific papers that can vary depending on the instructions of the journal. Usually, the Discussion section differs in length, shape, and structure, but it should be clear and brief [15–17]. Long, meandering text can distract so the structure provided can be used and subheading removed if they are not permitted by the journal. This is the main tip for writing the Discussion section. The first paragraph should give the main findings, which should follow to the result section of the Abstract, but removing the numbers and transforming the statistics into words, e.g., 50%, can be described as "half" in writing the results in words. The next paragraphs should cover strengths and limitations [18]. The latter should be written in a way so as to explain what the authors did to deal with the potential weaknesses and what limitations, if any, actually arise from them. After these deliberations, the authors should discuss their most important results comparing them with those of other similar published studies. Interpretation and implications of findings should be the final issue to describe before reaching the conclusion [19]. The conclusion section could be part of the Discussion or could be written separately, depending on the guidelines of the scientific journal. It should mirror the conclusion reached in the Abstract. Its conclusion must be in response to the study objectives set, but suggestions for future research and practice could be given too.

4.10 References

Each journal has its own instructions to follow regarding the style and the maximum number of references, explained in its instructions to authors in the journal website. All references should have the same style. References must be relevant and up-to-date. Consider key references from the last 5 years, depending on the subject.

Table 4.4 Suggested structure for the discussion section

- Statement of principal findings
- Strengths and weaknesses of the study
- Comparison with other studies in relation to strengths, weaknesses, and results
- Generalizability and implications of the findings for practice
- Lessons for future research

Careful management of the references is recommended because it could be a taken as indicator of the quality of the article [16]. The use of bibliographic managers can simplify and help. With many free softwares for management of bibliography, there is no excuse for not using them unless there are very references to cite.

4.11 Cover Letter

The cover letter can help introduce the work done to the journal editorial team, but nothing important for inclusion in the Introduction section of the paper should be delegated to the cover letter. Authors can use cover letter to highlight the significance of the research and to convince the editors that the research paper will make a good impact. However, it is the paper that will speak for itself; the cover letter cannot really replace good manuscript writing. Table 4.5 summarizes the common information included in a cover letter. It should be short, clear, and accurate. It should avoid humor and use a formal language. Each journal has its own rules; check if the journal's Instructions to Authors describe any cover letter requirements. In times when submission was via post and paper, the cover letter included a statement with the name of the journal's editor in chief, name of the journal, date of submission, and Title of the manuscript including the design of the study. A common cover letter structure was based on an introduction to the paper presented in one or two sentences; brief description of why the paper matched the specific journal's aims and scopes; summary of how the current study was valuable; confirmation from authors that the manuscript has not been published before and it is not in peer-review by another journal; and a declaration of who is the author to whom journal correspondence can be addressed. Note that many of these points are

Table 4.5 Information to include in a cover letter

Basic outline
– Editor's name
– Name of the journal
– Title of the manuscript
– Article type
– Brief background of the study and the research hypothesis
– Brief overview of the methods used
– Main findings and significant achievements
– Statement that the submission is not previously published nor currently under consideration by another journal
– Approval of all authors for submission of the manuscript to this journal
Other information commonly requested
– List of relevant studies by you or your co-authors that have been previously published
– Potential reviewers and their contact information
– If needed, reviewers to exclude
– Varied disclosures or statements required by journal (e.g., compliance with ethical standards, conflicts of interest, etc.)
– Compliance with reporting guidelines

frequently included in online forms filled when uploading the paper via a web-based portal, so including them in the cover letter additionally may be superfluous. Mix and match according to the journal's requirements.

4.12 Peer-Review, Response, and Resubmission

Peer-review has become a standard in medical journals as a means of attempting to preserve standards of academic publishing. The aim of peer-review is usually to help editors to decide if the manuscript is suitable for publication, permit critical feedback from experts (not necessarily anonymously), and improve the quality of the end-product. Although it has been demonstrated, peer-reviewed journals have better acceptance by clinicians [20], dealing with peer-reviewers is difficult for authors and needs guidance. Comments from editors and reviewers should be taken as attempts to improve the quality of the study. Suggestions made may not always be welcome or they may be misguided, but politeness at all times and a collaborative approach will be welcome by editors. After submitting a paper and following its assessment, a revision and a new resubmission may be required. This offer does not guarantee acceptance. Dealing with the revision task is not always easy. It needs proper attention to detail. There is no space for mistakes (a little hint of carelessness can lead to rejection). A weak, unelaborated answer to questions raised will render the article unacceptable, thus wasting an opportunity for success. The editor's letter requesting revisions would contain information about how to submit the revised manuscript, including instructions related to how to highlight the changes made and when the authors need to return the revised version. Please adhere to these. Use a tabulated form to answer to peer-reviewers' comment and be polite, brief, clear, and concise. It does no harm to the authors to thank to the reviewers and editors for their time and comments. Table 4.6 shows an example of an answer to peer-review. Respond to each point of each reviewer and numbering the issues highlighted by them with the answers and the changes made in the same row of the response table. This is the best way to clarify and to explain. A clean copy and a modified copy with the changes in a different letter color must be resubmitted in order to show what has been changed in the new resubmission. Ultimately if the paper is not accepted, it can be submitted elsewhere; there are many journals in any subject, and all papers ever written can end up being published as long as the author has perseverance.

4.13 Conclusion

Dealing with the process of publication of a new article can be stressful and an arduous task for any researcher. Being rejected is commonplace. It should encourage the author to revise and resubmit. The authors should take the reviewers´ comments as an opportunity to improve the quality of the paper. Experience and writing success

Table 4.6 Example of a structured answer to peer-review

Reviewer 1's comments		Author's response
	Abstract	
1	Page 1: Line 35: "SDM was reported in only 40%". This line is incomplete and should read "SDM was reported in only 40% of the studies"	We appreciate the suggestion. We have modified the text accordingly
	Introduction	
2	Page 2: Line 37–39: "Many authors have proposed personal strategies for promotion and practical application of SDM". The authors have quoted several references, however, should expand on different proposals on strategies and practical application of SDM	Thank you. We have added a paragraph explaining the different proposals as requested. The changes appear in the revised introduction section as follows: "A three-step model introducing choice, describing options, and exploring preferences has been suggested [10]. Another proposal involves encouraging patients to make their own care goals that clinicians translate into treatment plans [21]. Option grids and other decision aids are thought to make the SDM process easier. Measuring SDM as a quality indicator and reimbursing professionals that actually use SDM has been floated as another idea involving incentivization"
	Reviewer 2´s comments	
1	The results of the development of the tool and the advice of the experts should be presented in the results section and not in the methods section. The methods section only needs to state what we want to develop a new assessment tool, what methods to use, etc.	As the reviewer has requested, we have moved text from "2.3. Development of a quality assessment tool" from methods section to "3.2. Development of a quality assessment tool" in the revised Results section
2	Inclusion of exclusion criteria, the authors included CPGs and CSs about BC management, produced by governmental agencies or national and international professional organizations and societies, in other words, the exclusion of non-guidelines. So, it is not necessary to draft excluding randomized controlled trials (RCTs) and observational studies, narrative reviews, etc.	We have removed the text as advised.
3	Page 1, line 35, 139 + 28 = 167, please check thoroughly	We made the suggested modifications to the text
4	Page 1, line 37,42/101 = 41.6%. please check thoroughly	We have modified the text

don't have to go together. New authors can improve their chances of getting published by following the guidance in this chapter. Perseverance is the true name of the publication game.

References

1. Khan KS. The architecture of evidence-based gynaecology. Best Pract Res Clin Obstet Gynaecol. 2006;20(5):639–46.
2. Maes-Carballo M, Munoz-Nunez I, Martin-Diaz M, Mignini L, Bueno-Cavanillas A, Khan KS. Shared decision making in breast cancer treatment guidelines: development of a quality assessment tool and a systematic review. Health Expect. 2020;23:1045.
3. Kallestinova. How to write your first research paper. YALE J Biol Med. 2011;84:181–90.
4. Schulz KF, Altman DG, Moher D, Group C. CONSORT 2010 statement: updated guidelines for reporting parallel group randomised trials. Int J Surg. 2011;9(8):672–7.
5. Moher D, Hopewell S, Schulz KF, Montori V, Gotzsche PC, Devereaux PJ, et al. CONSORT 2010 explanation and elaboration: updated guidelines for reporting parallel group randomised trials. Int J Surg. 2012;10(1):28–55.
6. Liberati A, Altman DG, Tetzlaff J, Mulrow C, Gotzsche PC, Ioannidis JP, et al. The PRISMA statement for reporting systematic reviews and meta-analyses of studies that evaluate health care interventions: explanation and elaboration. Ann Intern Med. 2009;151(4):W65–94.
7. Moher D, Liberati A, Tetzlaff J, Altman DG, Group P. Preferred reporting items for systematic reviews and meta-analyses: the PRISMA statement. Open Med. 2009;3(3):e123–30.
8. Gallo V, Egger M, McCormack V, Farmer PB, Ioannidis JP, Kirsch-Volders M, et al. STrengthening the reporting of OBservational studies in epidemiology - molecular epidemiology (STROBE-ME): an extension of the STROBE statement. Prev Med. 2011;53(6):377–87.
9. Khan KS, Coomarasamy A. Searching for evidence to inform clinical practice. Curr Obstet Gynaecol. 2004;14(2):142–6.
10. Chien PF, Khan KS, Siassakos D. Registration of systematic reviews: PROSPERO. BJOG. 2012;119(8):903–5.
11. Martinez IA. Native and non-native writers' use of first person pronouns in the different sections of biology research articles in English. J Second Lang Writ. 2005;14(3):174–90.
12. Hofmann AH. Scientific writing and communication. Papers, proposals, and presentations. New York: Oxford University Press; 2010.
13. Rodman L. The active voice in scientific articles: frequency and discourse functions. J Tech Writ Commun. 1992;24(3):309–31.
14. Tarone LE, Gillette S, Icke V. On the use of the passive in two astrophysics journal papers with extensions to other languages and other fields. English for specific purposes. Engl Specif Purp. 1998;17:113–32.
15. Jenicek M. How to read, understand, and write 'Discussion' sections in medical articles. An exercise in critical thinking. Med Sci Monit. 2006;12(6):28–36.
16. Shokeir AA. How to write a medical original article: advice from an editor. Arab J Urol. 2014;12(1):71–8.
17. Faria Vieira R, de Lima RC, Gomide Mizubuti ES. How to write the discussion section of a scientific article. Acta Sci Agron. 2019;41:42621.
18. Coomarasamy A, Latthe P, Papaioannou S, Publicover M, Gee H, Khan KS. Critical appraisal in clinical practice: sometimes irrelevant, occasionally invalid. J R Soc Med. 2001;94(11):573–7.
19. Khan KS, Gee H. A new approach to teaching and learning in journal club. Med Teach. 1999;21(3):289–93.

20. Sievert ME, McKinin EJ, Johnson ED, Reid JC, Mitchell JA. Beyond relevance--characteristics of key papers for clinicians: an exploratory study in an academic setting. Bull Med Libr Assoc. 1996;84(3):351–8.
21. Maes-Carballo M, Munoz-Nunez I, Martin-Diaz M, et al. Shared decision making in breast cancer treatment guidelines: development of a quality assessment tool and a systematic review. Health Expect. 2020;23:1045. https://doi.org/10.1111/hex.13112.

Chapter 5
The Value of the Websites and Online Journals: The Modern Science

David Bloomer

Gutenberg changed the world; his development of printing in 1440–1450 ushered in a new form of mass communication that allowed ideas to be shared in a hitherto unprecedented way—and for over 500 years, its effectiveness was unsurpassed and the techniques it used surprisingly little changed. As late as the 1980s, many of the printing processes still widely used would have been consistent with the understandings of the original fifteenth-century pioneers of printing. Lead type was individually assembled and wedged into rigid frames, text corrections as minor as changing a simple comma could require laborious and time-consuming procedures by skilled craftsmen, and storage of typeset material would require massive volumes of lead to be shelved within heavy frames in large vaults (see Fig. 5.1 a, b).

It was a complex and labor-intensive procedure—and over the centuries equally time- consuming editorial processes were developed to ensure that the content, as well as the production, met high and exacting standards.

The whole process was regarded as both a craft and a creative art—and printers saw themselves as a pivotal to the dissemination of knowledge (see Fig. 5.2).

5.1 The Two Revolutions: In Production and in Distribution

Then came two revolutions, one following the other. Firstly, from the early 1980s onwards, the production process was progressively transformed by the digital revolution. Typesetting ceased to be a skilled craft requiring extensive inputs and industrial-type equipment. What had previously taken weeks to transform from

D. Bloomer (✉)
The Global Library of Women's Medicine, London, UK
e-mail: david.bloomer@glowm.com

G. C. Di Renzo (ed.), *Essential Writing, Communication and Narrative Skills for Medical Scientists Before and After the COVID Era*,
https://doi.org/10.1007/978-3-030-84954-2_5

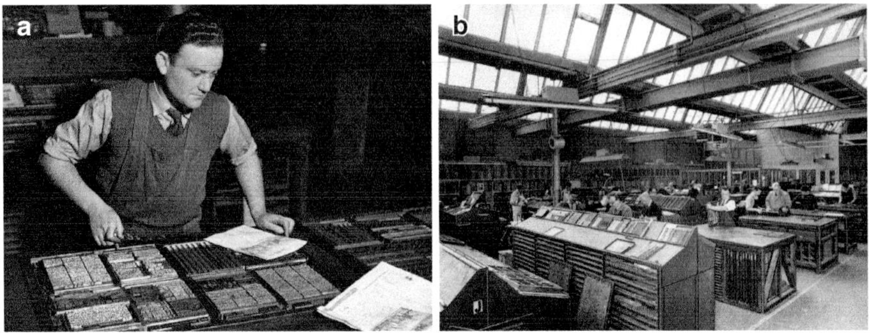

Fig. 5.1 (**a** and **b**) Before the digital revolution typesetting was a laborious and time-consuming skill requiring movable items of lead letters held together in heavy wooden frames. The advent of computer-based typesetting meant that up to a dozen skilled craftsmen working in large premises could be replaced by a single computer operator sitting at a desk—and taking a fraction of the time to achieve the same result

manuscript to type could now be done in hours, while corrections and textual changes that had previously taken hours could now be done in seconds. Even some of the editorial processes were streamlined as new programming instantly provided standard formats and error identification. Almost overnight anyone could create a typeset text and, thanks to basic photocopying techniques, could produce a quasi-published result.

Soon after this the second revolution occurred, when the development of the internet allowed a typeset text to be transferred to the other side of the world almost instantaneously. No longer did heavy reams of bound paper have to be shipped, via the world's normal cargo systems, to every destination; the text could be read by everyone everywhere instantaneously—provided, that is, they were part of the new internet network.

And for publishers, even the editorial processes were transformed. Manuscripts could be emailed by authors instead of mailed, proofs could similarly be sent out and author's corrections received—and so the whole editorial process, particularly in the field of science, was shortened dramatically. Publishing need no longer be a process involving many months but could be reduced to a few weeks or, even sometimes, days.

What is more it no longer even needed to involve publishers. Anyone could self-publish their own book, uplift it to the internet and hope that it would attract readers—some did and some did not, but many tried and still do. Their books may lack all the requirements of quality, accuracy of presentation, proper use of language, consistency of content, and literary standards that publishers set out to provide—but some audiences have not been deterred by such considerations.

So the advent of the digital age in the last years of the twentieth century fundamentally changed publishing. At the turn of the century, there was a widespread fear that the days of the conventional book were numbered—the brave new world seemed to herald the demise of conventional publishing.

THIS IS A

PRINTING OFFICE

CROSSROADS OF CIVILISATION

REFUGE OF ALL ARTS AGAINST THE RAVAGES OF TIME

ARMOURY OF FEARLESS TRUTH AGAINST

WHISPERING RUMOUR

INCESSANT TRUMPET OF TRADE

FROM THIS PLACE WORDS MAY FLY ABROAD NOT TO

PERISH ON WAVES OF SOUND, NOT TO VARY WITH

THE WRITER'S HAND BUT FIXED IN TIME,

HAVING BEEN VERIFIED BY PROOF

FRIEND, YOU STAND ON SACRED GROUND,

THIS IS A

PRINTING OFFICE

BEATRICE WARDE

Fig. 5.2 Traditional printing was a proud profession—a well-known sign that was often seen in printing offices

But to the relief of many, including traditional publishers of course, books are continuing to be published in great numbers and bookshops, although fewer still attract purchasers. In the UK, for example, the number of new printed titles published in 2018 (the most recent year for which statistics are available) was

184,000—but nevertheless there was a decline in sales income of about 5% from the previous year.

5.2 The Impact of Websites

Therefore, although traditional publishing has adapted and survived, in certain fields it has been overtaken—and in many circumstances superseded—by the worldwide reach, speed, and availability that the internet offers; this is particularly the case in medicine and other sciences where fast moving knowledge and up-to-date facts are at such a premium. The field of medicine is one where I have had long experience both as a conventional publisher and as a website publisher—and this field serves as a good example of a wider change.

5.2.1 The Time Factor

A typical clinical textbook in the field of medicine traditionally takes quite a long time to develop. Many such books feature a range of authors all writing separate chapters. But some of these authors typically complete their chapters before the others, indeed there may be up to a year between the first and the last—but the book cannot be published until all chapters have been completed. After that, allow 3–6 months for the actual production of the book and even on publication day some of the information in the book will already be nearly 2 years old. But it will remain on sale unchanged for, say, 5 years before a new edition may be produced.

As a result, readers are often presented with information that may be 7 or more years old—and in an increasingly fast-moving subject such as medicine that is simply no longer satisfactory. (Some publishers now try to ameliorate this problem by offering updates online—but this is not a very good or satisfactory solution.)

But publication of the same material on a website can transform this profile. Firstly, there is no need to wait for all the contributing authors to complete their chapters—each can be published as soon as it has been submitted and accepted. Secondly, the production process is much faster—perhaps 2 months as opposed to six. Thirdly, any chapter can be updated almost immediately whenever new information becomes available. Fourthly, the actual content of the publication can be enhanced by the use of video clips and animations that no conventional publication can ever offer. And finally, links can be included that offer almost instant access to other relevant information in other sources.

The result is a much more effective provision of knowledge transfer. Indeed, it is increasingly clear that wherever it is critical that knowledge is as up-to-date as possible conventional publishing will simply not be able to compete with internet-based, digital publishing. As a result medical websites have become very popular and widely used (see Fig. 5.3).

List of some of the most popular medical websites

1. PubMed	7. MedicineNet
2. Medscape	8. American Medical Association
3. WebMD	9. NIH
4. WHO	10. Epocrats
5. UptoDate	11. Mayo Clinic
6. ClinicalKey	12. NHS Direct

Fig. 5.3 Some of the currently most popular medical websites

That is not to say that printed material does not have some virtues—it is pleasant to use, it does not require any technological interface to view, and it is permanent. So for certain fields such as literature, history, or basic education, it should continue to have a valued place. But for science-based fields, conventional print publishing is likely to become largely redundant.

(As a footnote, it is perhaps worth noting, however, that the permanent nature of conventional printed publishing provides a particular virtue that digital publishing lacks; and while this may not seem important now it could become so in the future. Digital publishing depends on programming and technological equipment. But this can become obsolete—who now has the equipment to read a floppy disc or use a language program such as COBOL? Just a few years ago, they were standard, now they are forgotten. So in 100 or 200 years, how can we be sure that all our current digital files will still be accessible and readable? Printed books will be, of course).

5.2.2 *The Distribution Factor*

In the past, the traditional method of book distribution worked satisfactorily for those that lived in major population centers in the Western World—you visited a bookshop, you could browse through all the books they had in stock, and if they did not have a copy of the book you required, they ordered it for you and it would normally be available for collection within a few days. And this still works quite well for those people.

But, as any publisher will tell you, try and deliver books to many parts of the world, and it becomes very slow, very expensive, and very difficult—and for some locations almost impossible. Over many years, I attempted to arrange book deliveries to certain countries in parts of Africa, South America, and Asia and found it quite impractical. Even using courier services, where the cost of delivery could be twice as expensive as the book itself, failed to guarantee safe delivery.

So anyone living in vast swathes of the globe were penalized by a complete lack of access to new knowledge. In years gone by, I have personally visited the libraries of hospitals and medical schools in many African and some Asian countries and was frequently deeply saddened by the lack of access to good and up-to-date medical texts. A completely random collection of dusty volumes, maybe 30 or 40 years old, were often all that you could find. So traditional book distribution clearly failed in very many places, and the aspirations of many potential readers were undermined by lack of access.

And this is why internet-based, and more specifically, website-based, information has transformed knowledge transfer. Geography is no longer relevant, and your location in the world no longer determines your ability to participate at the highest level. In the sciences, perhaps particularly in the medical sciences, website-mediated information has proved the greatest possible contributor to advancement in understanding and practice. Quite simply, it has revolutionized the way we learn (see Fig. 5.4a, b).

Of course, there are many different kinds of websites fulfilling many different functions so that it is not feasible to make specific comments that can be applied usefully across the whole range. This chapter, therefore, focuses on educational websites in general and medical/scientific websites in particular. And I shall refer to the website that I manage not because it is special but because it provides relevant experience on which I can personally draw.

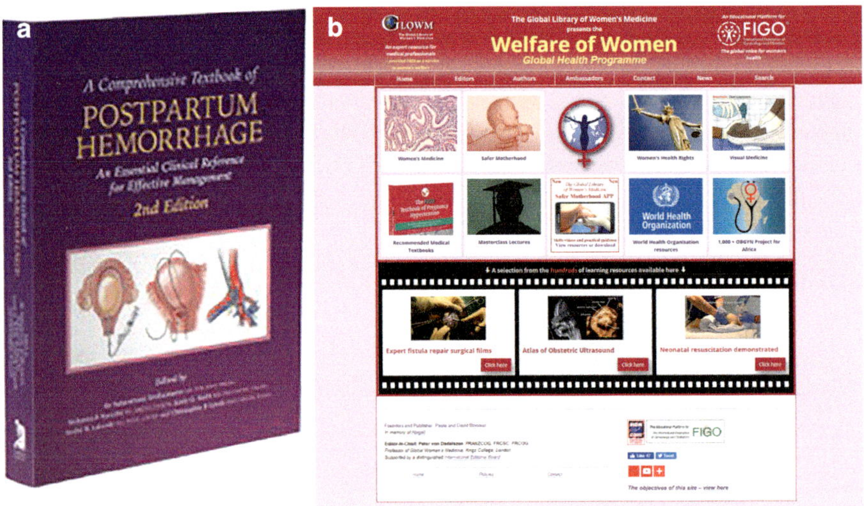

Fig. 5.4 (**a** and **b**) The traditional textbook is not only slow and expensive to produce but also relies for its distribution on a network of bookshops or on postal systems that are not universally available. Via a website multiple books can be made available instantly and at no additional cost anywhere in the world where there is an internet connection

5.2.3 *The Readership Factor*

Not only has the internet made it possible for websites to *speed up* communication in an astounding way—it has also meant that the *number* of people who are able to access this information has increased exponentially. Consider a simple clinical textbook on a medical topic—publishers used to be happy if it sold 2,000 copies or more worldwide over the course of its first 5 years (many sold less), and 10,000 copies sold was definitely a best-seller. Then compare this with the number of readers many good websites receive. *The Global Library of Women's Medicine*, to take one simple example from among many, currently receives some 400,000 visitors in a single month with up to 1,000,000 pages being viewed. There simply is *no* comparison in terms of readership and impact with a printed book.

Needless to say, some caution should be shown in comparing these figures—internet statistics are notoriously fickle and should be treated with considerable caution. Visitors usually include automatic bots that constantly search the internet, and also many of the people who visit a site may only stay on it for a very short time. But even after these considerations have been factored in the readership in 1 month vastly exceeds what a typical book might expect to receive in 60 months.

Furthermore, not only is the readership of any given text incomparably larger—but it is also incomparably wider. It reaches all corners of the world and all ranges of readers. In fact it democratizes knowledge in a way that was previously unthinkable. It also changes the way that learning is undertaken—no one source need be exclusively relied on. Increasingly, for example, students today are creating their own textbooks by taking chapters from different sources and building up their own tailor-made resource.

Finally, obtaining one's information from a website can, if it is well presented, be more effective and better explained than from a static printed text—the option of including videos, animated demonstration/diagrams and links to additional material make using this medium a much more dynamic experience than simply turning the pages of a printed text.

Only limited study has so far been undertaken to measure the true effectiveness of websites on scientific education [1]—but this is certainly a matter that deserves further study and analysis.

5.3 The Limitations to Website Knowledge Transfer and Future Developments

5.3.1 *The Availability of Satisfactory Internet Coverage*

Of course, there are still some limitations to the impact that websites can achieve. The most obvious of these is the current lack of universal internet coverage. Many parts of the world now have excellent internet coverage, but there are still large areas, principally in Africa and Asia, where this is not the case. In Africa in particular, very large areas are without effective coverage, and this can be a major disadvantage for those living there. For our part, we have tried to confront this problem by putting the whole of our very large website (thousands of text pages, over 30 hours of video presentations, elaborate visual atlases, etc.) onto small Memory Sticks which we then distribute to local "ambassadors" who download the whole website onto computers at the local hospitals and medical schools.

As a stop-gap measure this seems to have worked quite well. But it is only a stop-gap and cannot, of course, offer the constant updating that our normal website offers. So after a time, this whole process has to be repeated (which is costly and time-consuming) since otherwise this option loses its ability to guarantee reasonably current information and guidance.

5.3.2 An Alternative Solution

But there is an alternative solution. While the internet connectivity in Africa may still be very variable, unreliable, and poorly available, mobile phone connectivity is usually excellent and extensive—and covers very much more of the continent. In consequence, the possession of mobile phones in Africa is now almost universal (in fact in Kenya the majority of all financial transactions are done now via mobile phones). So this offers an alternative option that still makes reference to websites both feasible and useful.

Of course, with the current generation of smartphones, the size of the screens does limit the way that websites can be displayed and used—but they nevertheless are modestly practical alternatives. Currently, for example, in addition to our website we offer an app with many of our website resources on it, including complete textbooks, and these can be downloaded onto the phone so that they remain permanently available even when the phone is not within network connectivity. So short videos and illustrated texts can easily be viewed—and whilst no one would really want to read a full textbook cover-to-cover on a smartphone, it does at least offer an entirely practical way of accessing specific chapters or sections.

But the near future offers an even better possibility. Progress in technology never stands still, and this is particularly the case with communications technology. A few years ago, smartphones were a rare curiosity—now they are commonplace and standard. Today folding phones are only in their infancy and are just gradually and slowly being introduced. But within a few years, it is likely that they will be as widespread as smartphones are now. When unfolded their screens become small tablets (about the size perhaps of a typical paperback book when opened)—and this will make them entirely suitable for website viewing in a virtually normal way (see Fig. 5.5a, b).

Therefore, although nothing is certain, it seems very probable that folding phones will once again transform the way many people access and view information, and once again websites will gain an additional advantage over other options. So no longer will knowledge transfer be limited by the lack of internet connectivity.

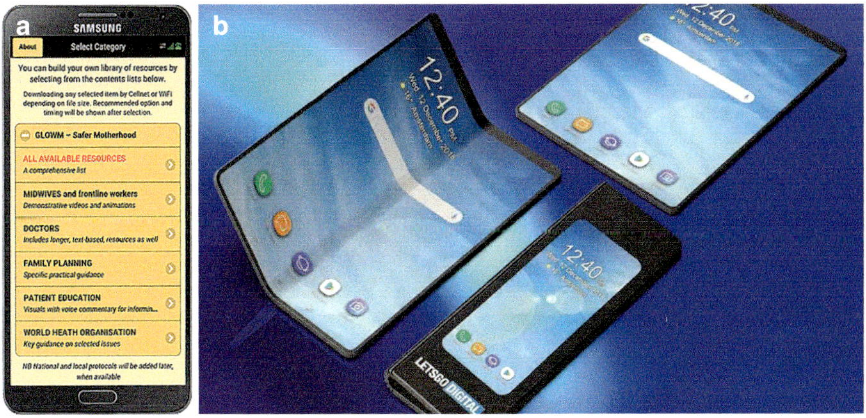
a
SAMSUNG
About
Select Category
You can build your own library of resources by selecting from the contents lists below.
Downloading any selected item by Cellnet or WiFi depending on file size. Recommended option and timing will be shown after selection.
GLOWM – Safer Motherhood
ALL AVAILABLE RESOURCES
A comprehensive list
MIDWIVES and frontline workers
Demonstrative videos and animations
DOCTORS
Includes longer, text-based, resources as well
FAMILY PLANNING
Specific practical guidance
PATIENT EDUCATION
Visuals with voice commentary for informin...
WORLD HEATH ORGANISATION
Key guidance on selected issues
NB National and local protocols will be added later, when available
b
12:40
LETSGO DIGITAL

Fig. 5.5 (**a** and **b**) Smartphones can currently provide practical information on their small screens and thus provide a useful alternative option where no internet connectivity is available. The large screens offered by the new generation of folding phones will transform this option by largely matching the visual detail available on laptop computers

5.3.3 Interactivity

But just as technology does not stand still, so websites will constantly need to evolve to meet the needs of their increasingly sophisticated users. Already they offer a wide diversity of presentational forms and experiences, but most of these are passive—the communication is in one direction only. It seems likely that this will change—users will demand more from their experience so elements of personalization and interactivity will increase. Already considerable steps have been made to personalize some websites to cater more specifically for user's needs, but, particularly in the field of learning, a more interactive experience will be demanded.

Of course this is likely to take many forms. As a tentative step into this field, for example, we (*The Global Library of Women's Medicine*) have just introduced the first 15 Volumes of an eventual 50 Volume Series of textbooks covering most aspects of women's medicine. And we are entitling these Volumes as being part of a *Continuous Textbook*, because every author of each chapter in every Volume will be able to *continuously* update his or her chapter whenever appropriate. These Volumes are also offering all readers an interactive option for *online learning assessment,* whereby readers will be able demonstrate that they have actually learned and understood what they have read by answering a range of multi-choice questions that will be provided at the end of each chapter.

Of course, this is only a modest start. But there is little doubt that as time passes increasingly more sophisticated ways will be developed to "involve" users of websites actively, thus giving them a more effective and pro-active experience from their learning activities.

5.3.4 *Language*

Another area that will require more attention and development if universal learning is to be truly enhanced relates to language. English is the principal language used for scientific research, which gives it a special advantage—but at a general educational level it is only one among many. In order to truly achieve effective universal communication, some answer is needed to this challenge—but it is not yet on the horizon. While Google and others have made bold steps by introducing translation programs, they are not yet able to provide sufficiently satisfactory results for any genuinely technical topic. Perhaps a combination of Artificial Intelligence and quantum computing may one day provide a workable solution—but this is certainly still seems to be some time away.

5.3.5 *Quality*

"GIGO"—garbage in garbage out—was a slogan coined in the early days of computer development, but it still applies today. It is one thing to have a website that provides information about important topics, but if it is not good and accurate then it fails to meet any worthwhile purpose. At the present time, there is no easy way to be certain that the website you are using meets the standards that you require. There are some validation systems that try to provide some minimal level of quality assurance but nothing that matches the peer-review system, for example, that scientific research journals apply. So, for the time being at least, website users must rely on their own judgment based on the qualifications of the website contributors, the standing and status of the organization that is producing it and the reputation it enjoys among other users. This is likely to change over time.

5.3.6 *Funding*

The traditional way of funding that supported conventional publishing over past times does not work with websites. Previously publishers produced books and if you wanted one you paid for it. But the internet provides such a vast raft of free information that an expectation has arisen that anything accessed on the internet will be free (although there are a range of exceptions to this, including online scientific journals).

Some websites do manage to charge for very specific services, but many struggle when they try to do so. As a result, various formulas have been developed to try and achieve financial viability. Advertising and sponsorship are two obviously possible options but both may have disadvantages too. Advertising can significantly undermine the reader experience and can act as a diversion—while sponsorship may raise concerns about impartiality unless it is undertaken carefully and transparently. So these are factors that will continue to be a challenge until more satisfactory and reliable funding options emerge.

5.4 Conclusion

But despite the various challenges that websites still face, any current disadvantages are massively outweighed by their obvious advantages (see Fig. 5.6).

Summarising the advantages and disadvantages of medical website,

in comparison to conventionally printed resources

Advantages	**Disadvantages**
Instant availability *Immediate and easy access*	Dependent on internet connectivity *Entirely ineffective where no adequate connectivity exists*
Range of content *Can include videos and animations in addition to text*	Not permanent *No record available once deleted or abandoned*
Never out-of date *Can be constantly updated*	No guarantee of quality *Poor standards of universally accepted quality control*
Allows interactive options *Enables user response and inputs*	Lacks some user flexibility *Screen requirement limits some user convenience*
Unlimited capacity *Unrestricted volume of information*	
Immediate cross reference access *Links provide immediate and easy cross referencing*	

Fig. 5.6 Summarizing the advantages and disadvantages of websites providing medical information

5.5 The Development of Online Journals

5.5.1 The Challenge of Documenting Scientific Advance in a Systematic Way

Scientific journals document the advances in scientific research around the world—and over the last century, the numbers have grown very rapidly [2]. No one is quite sure just how many peer-reviewed academic journals there are today, but it is generally believed that there are close to 30,000 and each year some three million papers are published in them. It is estimated that about 30% of these journals are in the biomedical sciences [3].

The number of papers in these journals continues to increase each year. So by any standards, a vast volume of new material is being generated annually and added to an already overwhelmingly large body of existing research data.

The description "peer reviewed" means that any paper published by a given journal has been subjected to review and approval by one or more (normally anonymous) experts who judge that it meets satisfactory scientific standards of probity, accuracy, and relevance. However, the descriptor "peer reviewed" can cover a range of quality standards, depending on the editorial policy of the journal in question. So, while it is a useful descriptor, it does not mean that every peer reviewed journal offers the same quality of assessment for the papers it publishes.

In order to provide a more precise indicator of a journal's scientific quality its "impact factor" within the scientific community is measured—this is an index that reflects the yearly average number of citations that articles published in the last 2 years in any given journal received. Once again, this does not guarantee that any individual article in a high impact journal may be scientifically more meritorious that one in a low impact journal, but it does reflect the fact that the scientific community on average takes more notice of papers in the high impact journal.

So neither the long-standing and important practice of peer-review nor the impact factor assignment provide absolute reassurances of scientific "quality" but they are as close as it is possible to get at present in providing some order and hierarchy to the vast quantity of research publications that are made available each year.

5.5.2 The Limitations of Conventional Publication

Traditionally, scientific peer reviewed journals have been published by a range of specialist publishers and also by some scientific societies and associations. And the publication process has been an extended one; for example it might take 6–12 months for a typical paper to be peer-reviewed, revised, re-reviewed, accepted, proofed, and printed. Then the journal still needs to be mailed to subscribers—and where they happen to be resident in different countries from the publisher this can also add a significant time.

While, therefore, a time gap of 12–18 months between the achievement of a scientific "finding" and its communication to other scientists was not disproportionately slow, given the necessary requirement of proper validation, its effective distribution to the scientific community was less than ideal because the numbers of readers it reached were so small. The physical number of copies printed and distributed of many journals was often in the region of 1000 copies or less (though some were much higher), and this often meant that the awareness of research results by those who might potentially be interested frequently depended on subsequent literature reviews that could easily take another year to be published and which were highly selective and variable in nature.

So the system that had evolved over very many decades for documenting and communicating scientific advances was essentially unstructured, somewhat random and difficult to navigate. The advent of online publication, however, has offered a major and highly significant improvement in the way that science is communicated and the way that relevant results are identified.

5.5.3 Why the Online Publication of Journals Has Changed the Way Researchers Work

Since the online publication of journals took off seriously in the 1990s, a fundamental change has taken place in the pattern of publishing. While not the most significant factor, speed has certainly increased considerably; partly, of course, this has been assisted by the use of internet communications throughout the editorial process in place of tediously slow postal communications—but more importantly because the pattern of publication has changed. No longer does a paper have to wait until the next monthly or quarterly issue of the journal is scheduled, it can be published online as soon as it has been approved and accepted and only later featured in the traditional contents list of a dated issue.

Little research has yet been done to compare the impact of online journals with that of simply printed ones [4], but there can be little doubt about the overall effects of this transition. Nearly all important scientific journals are now available online in one format or another.

So today, even if a journal still has a printed edition (and some no longer do), the relevance of this has greatly diminished. Where previously a publisher might have printed, for example, 1000 copies of a specialist journal today they might print only 100. And the publisher's most significant income does not come from selling those printed copies but from selling online subscriptions and, in particular, from selling downloads of individual papers to non-subscribers.

So while publication has certainly become significantly faster since online publishing was introduced, that is not the real reason why its advent has benefited the research community so greatly. It is the fact that the availability of most journals online has made the development of *search engines* possible that can almost instantly survey vast tranches of publications and topics and that therefore offer a pathway through the explosion of scientific data that is continuously being added to at an exponential rate.

There is just one other observation that may be relevant—and this relates to language. English is regarded as the fundamental language of scientific research so the vast majority of scientific journals are published in English. And this is the language used by nearly all the search engines when surveying the literature. But this means that much good research published in other languages may not get readily identified. This is a problem that still awaits a solution.

It also, incidentally, puts researchers who do not use or understand English at a significant disadvantage. Some journal editors make a special effort to help such researchers by assisting them in correcting their English to a sufficient level to be acceptable—but often this is not the case and so they are largely excluded.

5.5.4 Managing Quantity and Reducing Random Limitations

The increasing number of scientific research results being published in almost all areas of science has already been referred to and is widely understood. For any individual scientist, it has become almost impossible to maintain awareness of every new finding that might be relevant to his or her work—despite the existence of such reference aids as DOIs (Digital Object Identifiers) and ISSNs (International Standard Serial Numbers).

But the search mechanisms that are now available, and being constantly improved, make "literature mining" an invaluable new method of identifying relevant information across a vast field in a far more comprehensive way than the traditional, slow, and selective system of published reviews that were relied on previously.

A current example will serve to illustrate this well. At the time of writing, the world is suffering from the COVID-19 pandemic and scientists are working intensely to find answers. Each week currently, some 4000 new papers on the topic are being published, and a total of some 23,000 are now already available. It would therefore be quite impossible for any researchers using traditional survey procedures to keep properly abreast of all the new findings that might be relevant to their own special field of focus [5].

But the use of good search mechanisms makes this task much more manageable. Of course, this does depend on the quality of the algorithms used by the search engines. Academic search engines have now become the primary resource for scientists to turn to in order to find research papers and other scholarly sources. While classic academic databases like Web of Science and Scopus are locked behind pay walls, others such as Google Scholar can be accessed freely.

Google Scholar is perhaps the most frequently used search engine, and it covers approximately 200 million articles and, among other things, provides links to many of them. *Microsoft Academic* has similar coverage although its approach is somewhat different. Science.gov is distinctive in that it also offers free access to research results from 15 US Federal Agencies, while *CORE* focuses on Open Access research papers and *BASE* searches 130 million documents from over 6000 sources. *Baidu Scholar* is distinctive because although its interface is in Chinese its index contains research papers in English as well as Chinese—but perhaps of special note is *Semantic Scholar* because it uses algorithms powered by artificial intelligence in order to find hidden connections and links between research topics so that it can help to identify more relevant and impactful search results.

These, and a range of others, already fulfill a very worthwhile function in helping researchers locate relevant research, but one can anticipate that increasingly the application of *artificial intelligence* will be used in order to enhance the effectiveness of these automated search tools even further.

Related to this is the fact that big data analytics can also be called upon to extract meaningful patterns from the vast resources of facts and figures that the online availability of research results make available. Again, the current COVID-19 situation makes the point well—the extraordinary speed of advance in our understanding of the virus and of the development of vaccines and treatments which would normally be expected take years is now being attempted in months. In the age of conventional print publishing, no such attempt would have been conceivable.

An important development in recent times has been the movement towards "Open Access" publishing, which is having a profound effect on the publication of scientific research. The concept behind this movement is that research results should be freely available to all and not locked behind subscription and other pay walls. Particularly where research has been publically funded, it is suggested that it is inconsistent for the results to be copyrighted by commercial publishers or other organizations—thus restricting free access.

There are a number of different models of Open Access but basically the author of a paper, or the organization that funded the research, is required to pay for the quality control and other editorial processes involved in publication so that the research results can be made freely available to everyone.

This movement is developing very rapidly. In 2017, for example, it was reported that 13% of all research papers were already being published in "gold level" Open Access journals (i.e., the most complete form of open access) [6]. And 2019 some 12,500 Open Access journals (of all categories) were listed in *The Directory of Open Access Journals* [7].

There is no doubt that this movement will continue—and it does offer some obvious advantages and benefits, but it is not without some drawbacks. Most particularly whereas with a conventional journal the publisher pays all the publication costs with an Open Access journal, this burden falls on the authors of the paper. This is not a significant problem if the funders of their research agree to bear the costs, but where that is not the case, reseachers can only publish if they can afford the fees themselves.

It has also sometimes been suggested that making research results so universally available could lead to many more unqualified interpretations being presented that could serve to confuse and obfuscate proper discussion. Nevertheless, despite such reservations, it is clear that Open Access publishing will continue to grow although it is unlikely ever to completely supersede conventional publishing protocols.

There are other developments that are also likely to affect the publication pattern of scientific research journals—but nothing will match the impact that the introduction of online journal publishing is already having on the way scientific advances are communicated and understood.

5.6 The Catalytic Effect of COVID-19 on Scientific Publishing

As a final observation, it may be relevant to consider the potential effect that the COVID-19 pandemic is likely to have on scientific communication—just one, but a significant one, of the many long-term impacts that the epidemic will have on our future world.

It has become apparent during this epidemic that speed and personal interaction are now two increasingly central elements in achieving effective scientific advance. Where speed is important no longer is the traditional, printed word a satisfactory option. What we used to allow 10 or 15 years to develop, we are now trying to do in 10–15 months—as the current drive for COVID-19 vaccines demonstrates. And without the fact that most key research journals are now being published online, this would have been unthinkable.

Also, without the analytical power that enables intelligent search engines to identify and correlate key the research results that are now available online, it would also have been far less feasible. There can obviously be no turning back from these developments.

Personal interactions between specialist scientists, however, are also an essential element in this mix. Traditionally these have principally been undertaken via the many Symposia, Workshops, and Congresses that take place around the world. Not only is this method somewhat slow by modern standards, but the unprecedented "lockdown" of recent months has also made it impossible in practice by preventing nearly all travel.

Fortunately the internet has yet again come to science's aid and a wealth of opportunities have been created on a variety of different digital platforms (Skype, Zoom, Teams, and many others) to make immediate face-to-face meetings and discussion possible on a worldwide basis whether these are between 2 scientists or 100. Such options have proved effective, practical, easy-to-arrange, and popular.

There can be no going back from this. Traditional scientific meetings and congresses will certainly continue to be held once normal condition return, but they will be less numerous and less frequent. Increasingly these online digital platforms will be used for many such personal interactions and scientific debates. So we can confidently expect to see more scientific meetings, teaching sessions, and research symposia undertaken online, and we can also anticipate that many websites will also develop their profiles to incorporate some of the same features.

So there will be less expensive and time-consuming travel and many more less costly and faster specialist meetings online. Furthermore, the existing digital platforms that currently make such interpersonal meetings possible will be continuously developed and improved to greatly enhance the user experience involved. Within a few years, this online personal communication technology could become a new and very powerful catalyst for scientific debate, learning, and advance.

References

1. Thoma B, Sanders J, Lin M, Patterson Q, Steeg J, Chan T. The social media index: measuring the impact of emergency medicine and critical care websites. West J Emerg Med. 2015;16(2):242–9.
2. Mabe M, Amin M. Growth dynamics of scholarly and scientific journals. Scientometrics. 2001;51:147–62. https://doi.org/10.1023/A:1010520913124.
3. The STM report fifth edition October, 2018.
4. De Groote S, Dorsch J. Impact on print journal usage. Bull Med Libr Assoc. 2001;89(4):372–8.
5. Brainard J Scientists are drowning in COVID-19 papers. Can new tools keep them afloat? *Science Magazine* 13 May 2020 https://www.sciencemag.org/news/2020/05/scientists-are-drowning-covid-19-papers-can-new-tools-keep-them-afloat.
6. Crawford W. Gold open access 2013–2018: articles in journals GOA4) (PDF),2019. Cites & Insights Books. ISBN 978-1-329-54713-1.
7. Directory of Open Access Journals. https://doaj.org/.

Chapter 6
The Website Construction: The Door to Open Communication

Filippo Gruni

6.1 Introduction

During the lockdown period, I happened to run into a meme on Microsoft's well-known professional social network, Linkedin. The meme was a cartoon with the question "What was the force that triggered the digital change of your company?". Under the question, there were three options: "your innovation manager," "your desire for knowledge and improvement," and "the Coronavirus." This meme made me smile but also sparked a thought that matured day after day into the focal point of this chapter: how much has the lockdown experience changed us?

It is an inescapable truth that we have changed due to force majeure, or rather, a part of the world population (probably a clear majority) had to take a running start to shorten the distance between them and the younger generations and familiarize themselves with the digital tools of a communication that goes beyond time and space. This technological divide has undoubtedly participated in accentuating the generation gap.

Though the Coronavirus has objectively accelerated many companies and populations' digitization process, it hasn't revolutionized in any way the needs and the mechanics of communication. As psychologist Watzlawick's from the Palo Alto school rightly said: "We cannot not communicate." Let's explore how the actual communication needs of the professional and corporate world have changed, the strategies that can be used to generate empathy in a digital world where distance

F. Gruni (✉)
Lotrèk Digital Agency, Pistoia, Italy
e-mail: filippo@lotrek.it

G. C. Di Renzo (ed.), *Essential Writing, Communication and Narrative Skills for Medical Scientists Before and After the COVID Era*,
https://doi.org/10.1007/978-3-030-84954-2_6

reigns and time and space have disappeared and the ways in which we can make this flow of communication still human.

6.2 The Internet Revolution and Distance Communication

Imagine how overwhelmed the first passengers of slow steam trains must have felt as they travelled on the new railways of Europe. They sit motionless in their seats surrounded by narrow corridors and compartments, while they are hurtled away at a surprising speed. Their eyes are ensnared by a primordial virtual screen: the window. Images of real but distorted landscapes flow on this panoramic screen. The speed at which the train moves shows images of a terrain that has little to do with the real world.

It could be argued that the invention of the train had a clear influence on the way in which we observe the world. It has revolutionized the concept of space and time. Mankind was able to contract and bend it to suit its needs. The railway is but one example of nineteenth- and twentieth-century inventions that changed our perception of time and space. As Stephen Kern theorized in his 1983 essay: the telephone and the cinema did it and eventually so would television and, of course, the internet. Technology, therefore, is capable of revolutionizing the world as we know it, but we could also add that sometimes, profound societal changes are triggered by the unforeseen events that force us to adapt.

Although online communication had been part of our lives for a long time, the arrival and spread of COVID-19 accelerated its adoption and even at times managed to supplant our daily reality, even in situations people had obstinately considered only physical. Unsurprisingly, some undeterred supporters of offline communication found themselves catapulted into a world made up of rules and languages that were in some ways familiar, but in others completely different. Sociologist Domenico De Masi called it "total disorientation," but he further explains that the coronavirus health emergency is "a further step in a post-industrial society," where technology has made it possible to understand that "we are all in one great neighbourhood where things resonate quickly."[1]

The Internet is certainly not a recent invention (and neither are tools like webinars), but its main function, the ability to connect or, as the name suggests, create a *network*, is being rediscovered. We can connect the two inventions of the railway and the internet through Manuel Castelles' definition of the space of information flows which is different from the physical one. But just like it, it is made of networks, junctions, lines, and stations, where territorial distances are measured through virtual proximity. In the COVID-19 era, the internet certainly hasn't been completely able to erase spatial distances (it would have been too much to expect),

[1] https://www.ansa.it/sito/notizie/tecnologia/tlc/2020/02/27/de-masi-coronavirus-esperimento-tech_6c904ef1-e13c-4330-8cf5-d436a4c1adc2.html

but it has – as Tiziano Bonini claims – mediated them; that is, digital media have "profoundly changed the field of interpersonal relationships at a distance."[2]

Online communication doesn't play out as it would in a real environment since physical distance can never be truly set aside. The lack of proximity between the speaker and the listener makes the use of technological tools, like computer or smartphone webcams and microphones, necessary. In every interaction, there is always something that stands between two or more participants. These technological tools aren't always familiar to everyone, and the initial lack of knowledge can accentuate problems such as delays, misunderstandings, and difficulties in hearing or seeing well. In a sense, communication mediated by a device is somewhat imperfect and maybe this characteristic makes it a little more human.

The non-verbal and para-verbal cues which sustain speech and help us interpret our interlocutor's message are often missing in distance communication. Simple things such as facial expressions, posture, and intonation are absent in written communication. We must resort to "smilies," extra punctuation marks, abbreviations, and other conventions which would not be tolerated in other written interactions.

As previously mentioned, one of the many advantages of mediated communication is the ability to go beyond the limits of space and time. Two people on opposite sides of the world can now communicate through emails, video conferences, and messaging apps. The last two were greatly used during the lockdown because they gave the possibility to communicate in real time. Technically speaking, we divide distance communication into two categories: asynchronous and synchronous communication. An email, for example, is asynchronous, because the reader and writer see it at different times (deferred). Oppositely, a video conference is synchronous. The users are connected and communicate in real time. Compared to face-to-face communication, distance communication tools make it possible to obtain messages that survive the test of time but can also be modified and adapted.

There are two further differences between face-to-face and online communication. One is linked to the lack of feedback, the other to the identity of the participants. In some cases, the non-verbal cues of the listener can serve as positive or negative feedback, but the very nature of distance communication can cause a message to receive a delayed response. When it comes to identity, the virtual world lends itself to redefining the participants' roles. At times, the fact that they can hide behind nicknames makes them more likely to express themselves without fear.

This "alter-ego" identity can be a double-edged sword, but with the spread of virtual communities, the online world has created its own etiquette of rules and conventions designed to guarantee the correct and compliant behaviour of its users. The technical term is netiquette, a combination of net and etiquette.

Despite some limitations, online communication has not only become more immediate but also an essential tool for our daily activities, especially in the workplace. Sending and receiving written, audio, or video messages remotely is at the

[2] T. Bonini, *L'immaginazione sociologica e le conseguenze sociali del Covid-19,* in Mediascapes journal 15/2020

heart of our daily communication, from training to marketing. Marketing is now considered by many as synonymous to web marketing: an online strategy to reach people interested in the products or services that a company offers.

While advertising flyers have morphed into sponsored social media content to reach a wider audience, physical events and meetings have also found their virtual counterpart with webinars. This tool, translated as an "online seminar" (from web-based seminar), has multiple potential uses and, although it has been within the reach of many for several years, is going through a renaissance in this period of social distancing.

6.3 Continue to Communicate: From the Physical Event to the Webinar

The MICE industry (an acronym for meetings, incentives, conferences, and exhibitions) is a world where an infinite number of work sectors intersect. This industry creates an incredible amount of satellite activities, events animate places and move people and therefore money, but also have the ability to make ideas and knowledge circulate. In extraordinary situations like the lockdown, people can travel on other channels, without having to completely stop. Of course, the persons employed in this industry and the ones connected to it have suffered substantial losses, but these recent times have also encouraged many agencies to adapt. In the long run, the ones that have worked the hardest to grow gills will survive best in this sea of change.

What happens, however, when the physical meetings, the handshakes, the round table discussions at the basis of these events, cease to exist? Do events lose all their meaning or does something remain? When a "physical" event is no longer actually feasible, does an underlying essence endure? Yes, and it is the need, if not the goal, to communicate something, be it a company's new discovery, the launch of a new product, or a brand's new line.

6.3.1 Why a Webinar

If almost all companies, institutions and professionals have poured rivers of webinars online during this COVID era, it wasn't only because of an urgent desire to feel closer to others, but also because evidence spread that this tool can be much more than just a remote seminar filled with boring slides.

A webinar is an online meeting made possible through a video conferencing software, which, however, allows for considerable interaction between the speakers and sometimes also the users. Usually, a webinar uses a one-to-many communication style. One or a few speakers address an audience connected online that listens but can also be asked to interact. Even when it comes to a lecture-style webinar, the speaker can make use of additional tools such as screen-sharing to illustrate their ideas through slides and videos. In cases when webinar participants are expected to engage more, features can be activated to encourage participation. Some webinar organisers opt for a chat where users can make comments or ask questions and then receive a live answer (which benefits the whole group), others use it as an opportunity to launch studies and surveys or to collect data from participants through forms. The collected data could later be used for email marketing (sending promotional emails) or Customer Relationship Management operations (maintaining a good relationship with customers).

The use of the webinar is at least a decade-old, but over that time period, it has adapted to various contexts and to the evolution of technologies and marketing objectives. One of its most common purposes is training. Webinars were originally created to disseminate educational information to the public, be it the internal team of a company that has to receive on-going training or potential customers interested in a new version of a product. There are many ways to communicate content: these range from no participant involvement in a lecture-style webinar (typically used for lessons and courses) to mild participant involvement through chats and writing tools, all the way to the active involvement of multiple speakers or even the listeners themselves, using the support of a moderator who can also act as a director.

Reaching one's audience everywhere has obvious advantages which pushed a wide range of professionals to test webinars during the lockdown. Many used this tool to provide courses and training (of varying levels of validity) that physical distance had interrupted. Others used webinars to analyze the current situation, for example, government bodies and institutions illustrated data and forecasts in a video format or gave insights to essential sectors on how to cope with the difficulties they were encountering. Last but not least, companies understood the potential of webinars as a marketing tool. People were suddenly spending much more time at home, and it, therefore, became easier to interest them in learning something new, discovering the secrets of a product, or finding answers to their questions directly from their computer.

6.3.2 The Fundamentals for a Successful Webinar

Packing suitcases, catching planes, booking hotel rooms, choosing the right catering for the countless coffee breaks, selecting a location, and networking at aperitifs are but some of the crucial details event organisers have to face. One look at this list and a less experienced person might think the webinar option is far simpler to organise, and since everything is virtual, the exhausting attention to detail becomes superfluous. Nothing could be more wrong, a webinar requires the careful planning of an infinite number of elements, and any form of improvisation should be banned.

Even if in some cases and in certain contexts the webinar can become a substitute for a physical event, one should consider how the message might change to adapt to the choice of communication medium. As sociologist McLuhan said "the medium is the message."

The first step of online event organisation is to identify a target audience and build a narrative that meets well-defined needs. It will therefore be necessary to prepare a detailed outline, perhaps accompanied by a storyboard that helps to predict the various video moments and takes. The storytelling technique can be a valuable aid to communicate something, even for commercial purposes. Because webinars are similar in nature to a televised event, choosing a charismatic moderator, who knows how to maintain the audience's attention is a good idea. Equally, using accompanying videos and slides, (as long as they are brief and graphically appealing) can help keep participants engaged. If event organisers are familiar with their target audience, they can choose the appropriate technology, the most suitable platform and also anticipate any problems that may arise for the participants who are not familiar with these means of communication.

Even though distance communication clearly reduces the presence of non-verbal elements, maintaining a certain tone of voice, paying attention to gestures, posture, and even clothing remains important. Just like in a physical event that involves different people, it is good practice to follow some rules for online communication, or netiquette, that regulates the terms and methods of participation of the speakers, manages well their allotted times and interventions.

Finally, in the marketing world, there is a recurrent mantra "content is king" that emphasises the fundamental importance of content which should never be taken for granted. A good webinar, just like a good post on social media or on a blog, must first and foremost have valid and useful content, which enriches, entertains, and interests the recipient on the other side of the screen.

6.3.3 The Main Webinar Platforms

Therefore, designing a quality webinar constitutes an investment in terms of authority, time, but also money, since monthly or annual subscription formulas allow organisers to have advantageous personalized platforms, whose cost undoubtedly differs from the one of a physical event.

The choice of the platform, like all the other details, should not be left to chance, because it affects the impression the participants have of the company or whoever holds the webinar. A decision must be made on the basis of the platform's features. Does it give the possibility to share information or the screen? Does it have a chat or a specific section for questions to the speaker? But above all, does it respect the communicative needs of the organizers of the digital event?

So what are the best video conferencing software tools to hold a webinar out on the market?

6.3.3.1 Demio

Demio is a platform that hosts up to 500 participants and is geared towards selling products through live-streaming events. This is the reason why it offers features that facilitate continuous interaction with participants (chats, surveys, and event reminders), environmental branding, and the collection of performance indicators.

6.3.3.2 WebinarNinja

Demio's main competitor when it comes to conversions on the customer journey, it is an excellent choice to push the consumer to take actions that will then lead to a sale. It differentiates itself from other platforms by giving the possibility of integrating over 1000 apps through Zapier, a tool created to automate various online processes. WebinarNinja gives the possibility to hold four types of events: in addition to live streaming, there are also recorded webinars, series, and a hybrid formula. It can host up to 1000 participants, with one or more speakers.

6.3.3.3 WebinarJam

WebinarJam is another platform worth mentioning in the world of webinars orientated toward sales promotion. In addition to being the simplest platform to use for those who have never created a webinar, it allows the user to insert pop-ups for the direct sale of a product during the event. The software also provides integrations with the main social media platforms. The webinar can also be seen in live-streaming directly on Youtube by inserting a password. This is a decisive feature, particularly for those who want to give more visibility to their event on social media.

6.3.3.4 GoToWebinar

GoToWebinar has proven itself as a solid platform capable of maintaining a stable connection which makes it the ideal solution for companies more interested in delivering rich content than the explicit promotion of a single product or service. It lends itself perfectly to content marketing operations, a strategy where useful content, linked to users' areas of expertise, is provided in order to attract them to a specific brand. It is the same system some companies use when they start a blog or publish short videos on social networks like Instagram. GoToWebinar also automatically records live webinars and allows the webinar creator to subsequently send the recording. On the downside, it does not offer particularly detailed marketing features.

6.3.3.5 CiscoWebEx

CiscoWebEx's most distinguishing feature is the shared whiteboard, which allows the users to make modifications synchronously. This feature makes the platform interesting from an educational or co-creation perspective since it makes one-to-one, as well as direct communication, possible. Brainstorming is no longer a problem, even if the members of the workgroup are miles away.

6.3.3.6 Zoom

Born as a platform for video conferencing (the Italian version was released in June 2020), it is the best software in terms of quality price on the market. Up to 100 participants can connect in audio and video with the basic version. The webinar can be simultaneously broadcasted on Facebook Live and Youtube with an unlimited number of participants. In addition, it features control tools, such as the ability to mute a participant or manage speaker turns. It also has other useful tools such as a whiteboard, note taking tools and the possibility to give participants an entrance test prior to the event.

6.4 Webinars as a Marketing Tool

The webinar is a perfect link between the world of business and the one of education. As previously mentioned, a webinar is an online video conference between one or more speakers and an audience, potentially made up of people from around the world. These people will be given a chance to learn more about a particular theme, product, or service and interact in the digital world.

If companies want to keep up with the developments in digital marketing, they clearly need to include webinars in their basket of services. At this point, let's focus on understanding why and how this tool can become one of a company's marketing strategy pillars or more specifically how webinars can help convert a user from a potential buyer to a customer, preferably a loyal one.

In fact, the purpose of a webinar is to convince a customer to consider the idea of getting in touch with a product or service provider. Companies can encourage potential clients to trust them by providing quality content, showing a high level of competence and becoming an authority in their target audience's sector of interest.

The webinar tool therefore belongs to the vast universe of content marketing, with which the traditional sales path is revolutionized: it is no longer the producer who seeks the consumer, but the opposite. The consumer is no longer bombarded with product advertisement, but rather, attracted to the brand through the company's use of quality content, especially when presented in an impartial way. The objective is to educate before selling. Webinars are the perfect medium to present a company's philosophy, values, and products and establish a connection with the audience.

Based on the previously mentioned points, it becomes extremely clear that webinars offer many benefits. In addition to significant savings in terms of organizational costs, webinars allow a company to get in direct contact with the target group its initial analysis has identified for a marketing campaign. The interactivity provided by webinar platforms through features such as chats, polls, and call-to-actions potentially transform the one-to-many communication of traditional videoconferencing into one-to-one communication. Through constant dialoguing and listening, companies can get to know their target audience, gain related cultural insights, and increase the level of user involvement both quantitatively and qualitatively.

Another non negligible advantage is the webinar's "2-in-1" formula: it is possible to reach your target group in two distinct moments, at first, during the live "broadcast" and then successively by making its recording available as a free video resource, usable in its entirety or by extracting its more significant clips.

Furthermore, webinars are a powerful tool for generating new leads, especially if filling an online form is required to participate. The term lead is used whenever a company encourages a user to give out his/her personal information through some form of marketing action. This information can then be used in a sales optic to contact the user. The most coveted data is definitely the email address, which is why webinars have a double strategic value for both content marketing and email marketing.

The generated leads are usually good because participant motivation is very high: those who decide to register and then participate in a webinar, even if also partly attracted by the free offer, show a much higher level of interest in the company and in the topic treated during the webinar than those who download, for example, a simple pdf guide. This is because the effort they devote to participate in a webinar is greater than the one required to take advantage of other types of free resources.

"Content is the king, but distribution is the queen and she wears the pants."[3] Though it is true that a webinar is a great means to produce and convey quality content, it will all come to nought if a company can't distribute it effectively. The key to a successful online event is promotion: on the company's own social media channels or on the ones owned by testimonials and endorsers. Surely, however, the most effective tactic is to use the user's email, initially as an invitation and to share information, and later, as a reminder both to those who have decided to sign up and to those who are still doubtful.

If a company chooses to use social networks, its own follower base is a good place to start, as long as those users are actually interested in what is offered. They are considered as being part of the target audience if they match the typical customer profile that is being targeted. Posts are a good tool to reveal the webinar's date and content and, for companies that use Facebook, a way to create a personalised event, where updates can be published to drum up interest for the event. The main social media platforms offer the possibility of giving more visibility to company's

[3] Jonathan Perelman, BuzzFeed

content through paid personalised promotional campaigns. Small groups of users, interested in a particular subject, are also a good place to find potential participants for a webinar.

Furthermore, websites, the company's shop window, should never be neglected. A user could enter the website (e.g., to look for a product) and be attracted by the news of an upcoming webinar. Blogs are also a good place to publish an article that anticipates the subjects covered in the seminar. A banner on the homepage or a pop-up that invites users to register are also a good means of gathering participants.

If a company already possesses a list of newsletter subscribers, it can promote the webinar there and include a registration form for interested participants. That way, the users will automatically receive a reminder before the online event starts. Of course, all these steps must be made in compliance with the regulations on the processing of personal data.

Last but not least, companies can rely on aggregator websites that offer a program of scheduled events divided by category. One of the most renowned ones is EventBrite, which in addition to hosting physical events gives space to virtual events such as webinars. This platform offers advantages such as reminders, to keep subscribers apprised of an upcoming event, but also the possibility to purchase a ticket should the organiser decide to charge an entry fee for the webinar.

6.4.1 Webinar Security and Privacy

The expression "collection of personal information" immediately brings to mind questions about privacy, security, and GDPR. The processing and management of sensitive data by online platforms, whose conditions of use, or pseudo-contracts through which privacy conditions, and rules of conduct are defined, are becoming increasingly more opaque due to a lack of supranational legislation.

In order to strengthen the protection of the personal data of its citizens and residents, the European Union has legislated on the subject by implementing the General Data Protection Regulation, better known as GDPR, starting from May 2018.

Since webinars are an integral part of web marketing strategies, it is important to remind organisers of their duties and the practices they should follow regarding the management of sensitive and personal data.

The changes introduced by the GDPR can be condensed into three main sections which are assigned to the company's legal representative in his/her position as data controller:

- The collection of personal data must be relevant to a specific purpose. The list of *prospective customers* and related data must be regularly cleaned and reviewed for each new marketing activity plan in order to have the user's consent for that particular marketing activity. Furthermore, the data retention period corresponds to the time necessary for the purposes for which it was collected.

- The burden of proof passes to the companies, which, in the event of disputes, must be able to demonstrate that they have complied with the legislation on the collection and processing of personal data.
- The company must undertake the mandatory training of employees in terms of security and privacy, in order to avoid improper or incorrect use of personal data outside of the permitted processing purposes.

When it comes to lead generation, one of the typical purposes of a webinar, the event organiser must give participants appropriate information, get consent to the processing of their personal data, and give them the possibility to refuse future business contacts at any time.

The security of webinars is also an important aspect to consider. These online events are often subject to threats, such as the hacking of the admin account, theft, which could result in the dissemination of sensitive data, or bombing, which is an interruption of the event with inappropriate videos or images.

Here are some tips to follow in order to avoid unpleasant situations[4]:

- Establish access systems and times to the virtual room.
- Define roles and privileges.
- Provide access codes.
- Maintain control of audio and video during the live stream.
- Make sure the recording of the conference is encrypted.

6.5 Conclusions

In conclusion, we can say that the webinar tool has a dual purpose; it can be used both as a marketing tool and as a functional one.

The perfect choice for a project on a larger scale that is both informative and commercial is a webinar platform that offers extra features such as emailing, the creation of a landing page for event registration and the collection of contacts into mailing lists that can later be used for newsletter activities.

On the other hand, when the objective is disseminating content, informing, and responding to the needs of a community, structured platforms for web conferences like Zoom are a simpler and more suitable option.

Undoubtedly, regardless of the platform used, being able to overcome the limitations of space and time will certainly grant companies access to a wider audience. Though webinar platforms will probably suffer a decreased rate of engagement due to the most basic of human dynamics: the easier and more immediate the access to content is, the weaker its impact on those who use it will be, I am still convinced that moving a company's presence online can only be beneficial.

[4] https://cdn2.hubspot.net/hubfs/437762/Takeaway_documents/Security_White_Paper-Final.pdf

Chapter 7
Ways to Implement Scientific Communication in the COVID-19 Era and Beyond

Gian Carlo Di Renzo, Valentina Tosto, Valentina Tsibizova, Khalid Saeed Khan, and Shehnoor Azhar

7.1 Introduction

Pandemics have no known boundaries [1]. Whether it was medieval plague that ravaged continents or malaria that continues to bite in significant numbers, the quest to find an equitable global health system continues. The history of pandemics also traces the origin of discipline of public health rooted in centuries-old concepts of hygiene and sanitation that continue to be the dominant theme despite enormous global burden of non-communicable diseases discovered in past few decades or so. The practice of quarantine was institutionalized to keep bubonic plague from reaching shores at various ports of entry. It was mandatory for the arriving crew and merchandise to wait for 40 days on ships before they could disembark.

G. C. Di Renzo
Department of Obstetrics and Gynecology, Centre of Perinatal and Reproductive Medicine, University of Perugia, Perugia, Italy

V. Tosto
Department of Obstetrics and Gynecology, IM Sechenov First State University, Moscow, Russia

V. Tsibizova
Almazov National Medical Research Centre, Health Ministry of Russian Federation, Saint Petersburg, Russia

K. S. Khan
Department of Preventive Medicine and Public Health, Faculty of Medicine, University of Granada, Granada, Spain

S. Azhar (✉)
Public Health University of Health Sciences, Lahore, Pakistan

University of Granada, Granada, Spain

G. C. Di Renzo (ed.), *Essential Writing, Communication and Narrative Skills for Medical Scientists Before and After the COVID Era*,
https://doi.org/10.1007/978-3-030-84954-2_7

Ever since unhygienic lifestyles and unsanitary civic conditions of the past were discovered as predisposing factors of infectious diseases like measles, yellow fever, and smallpox, diseases that shaped major political upheavals in the Americas and Europe, tremendous strides have been made in applying a scientific lens to prevention and control of infections. Enormous resources, both human and financial, have been spent in understanding microbiological phenomena in context of its transmissibility in each environment. Similarly, numerous administrative codes and sociocultural norms been institutionalized as evident in stringent health-related travel advisories seen today. Notwithstanding the miraculous accidental discovery of Penicillin that raised hopes for ending microbial infections, the fight turned out to be far from over in fact turning into much complex challenges to date as represented in antibiotic-resistant bacteria, emerging viruses and virions, and opportunist fungi.

The twentieth-century paradigm of infectious diseases beginning from Penicillin discovery is also noteworthy for the rise of evidence-based infectious disease management that shaped commercialization of anti-microbial agents relying on expansion of experimental laboratories in the industrialized world [2]. It was the beginning of a remarkable success stories that made various antibiotic medications household names. Newer products and formulations resulted in reducing the higher burden of hospital-acquired infections hence the quality of care and clinical outcomes. It was probably not until the high case fatality rate of 1994 epidemic of *Vibrio cholerae* 01 El Tor in Rwandan refugee camps that red flags were raised [1]. The causative microbe had appeared in different small-scale outbreaks worldwide throughout the twentieth century, but 1994 cholera outbreak was the first real awakening to the threat fueled by overuse of antimicrobial drugs. The advent of more virulent and infective bacterial species opened a new frontier calling for a global response to restrict this outbreak that resulted in several hundred thousand deaths within a very short period. World Health Organization of that period took the lead in gathering its global resources to constitute a multinational taskforce that advised to finally overcome that deadly outbreak. Internet connectivity was introduced around the same time.

Global connectivity has been underutilized to control the ongoing COVID pandemic mainly due to underpreparedness and even unpreparedness [3]. Despite viral outbreaks since the turn of this century known as Middle East Respiratory Syndrome (MERS), Severe Acute Respiratory Syndrome I (SARS 1), and Ebola Virus Hemorrhagic Fever (EVHF), the contrast with 1994 Vibrio cholera outbreak is stark considering the availability of digital tools and information sharing platforms available today. It could be argued that the challenge posed by the novel coronavirus is far bigger owing to its transmissibility via asymptomatic carriers, limitations of medical diagnostics, and anthropogenic factors that disrupt ecosystems at a far greater scale [3, 4].

In the hindsight though, the implications of three earlier outbreaks on international travel, commerce, and economy should have been better documented in public health literature. Lessons learned from previous episodes should have better passed on to the younger generation of health workers and public health workforce to prepare them for a more coherent response to a COVID-like scenario. It does not seem likely for historic technological and digital gulf that divides the global North and South will shrink anytime soon either. Does it mean to harness potential of omnipresent cellular networks and digital communication across continents more effectively to deliver a multinational response to any future pandemics modelled on 1994 El Tor outbreak? The answer is likely in affirmative due to effective care models of e-health and m-health rolled out elsewhere for delivering an array of health services be it road safety measures in Latin America, or maternal, neonatal, and child health in Afghanistan.

Communication technology is a vital tool that must be utilized effectively for complete control of the current pandemic and as bulwark against future ones. The dual threat of novel viruses and antibiotic-resistant bacteria pose formidable challenges to lifestyles and economies particularly in low-and-middle-income countries (LMICs) where the burden of non-communicable disease is already disproportionate. Amid weak public health infrastructure in LMICs that seem unlikely to attract public funding in short-term, a global re-orientation of priorities could help LMICs reach out to communities within their territories and beyond. Within available digital footprint worldwide, high-income countries (HICs) must be encouraged and incentivized by the entities like WHO, to institutionalize a meaningful engagement with LMICs for with the aim to prevent and respond to future health emergencies. Already, emergence of "frontline researchers" and "non-pharmaceutical interventions" (NPI) worldwide have generated enormous public interest in health topics, possibly a silver lining or a legacy of the ongoing emergency.

7.2 Avenues of Scientific Communication

In this chapter, scientific communication has been aimed at masses and at clinical staff with public health professionals straddling both groups as a common areas in any Venn Diagram. What separate the two groups is the freedom enjoyed by masses to choose their sources of health information and education, while healthcare professionals and clinicians are bound by clinical protocols derived from scientific evidence even if in a foreign setting.

Before November 2019, a health information and communication equilibrium existed (Fig. 7.1) since last reported pandemic of Spanish Flu nearly hundred years ago. When SARS-CoV-II cases started to pile up, a melee in healthcare was witnessed in both developing and developed world [4]. Underestimation, lowered threat perception of contagion, and shortages of personal protective equipment resulted in tens of thousands healthcare workers worldwide paying the ultimate price. One estimate suggests the number to be over 100,000. The state of clinical care was no different since obscured pathophysiological pathways blinded both diagnostics and treatments. Despite rapid genome sequencing in state-of-the-art laboratories within weeks of coronavirus detection in Wuhan (China), there were almost no definitive pharmaceutical solutions in sight. In fact, the term "non-pharmaceutical interventions or NPIs" gained traction and possibly remains most in the public memory since the pandemic began. Concurrently, extensive media

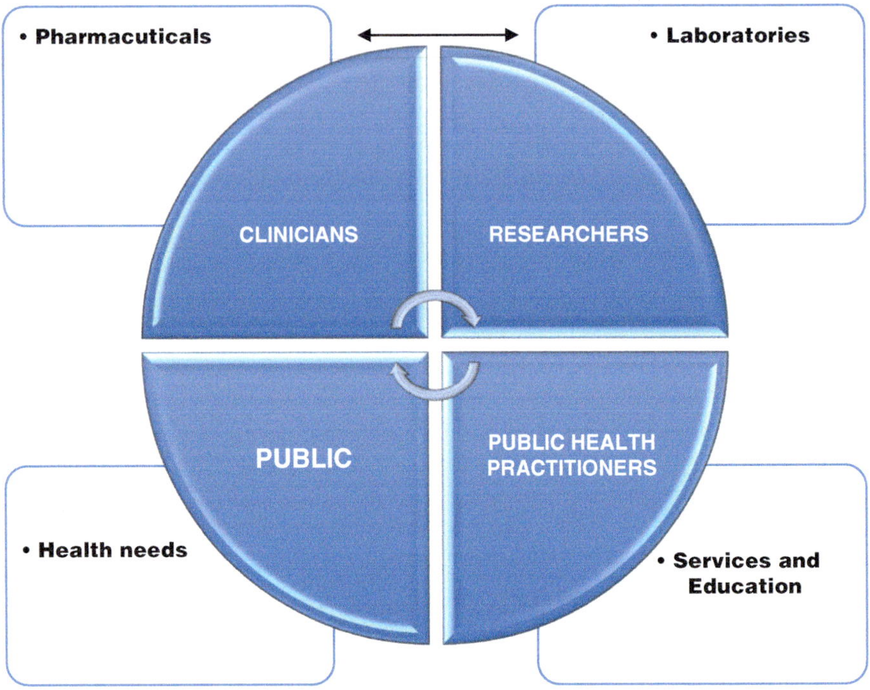

Fig. 7.1 Interrelationship of various communication actors in a health continuum

reporting on Emergency Use Authorizations "EUAs" of various candidate vaccines have made their manufacturers household names. Both vaccines and vaccinations have emerged prominently in public's consciousness as distinct causes set to alter the political economy of healthcare worldwide. By mid-2021, a slew of candidate vaccines are undergoing Phase III clinical trials across the world, while those granted EUAs during 2020 are set to get regular commercial approvals from regulators that from Food and Drug Administration (FDA) being the most sought after.

The disturbances of traditional communication equilibrium are significant in having once again confirmed the widespread influence of the old-school cable news cycle as the key source of health information [2, 4]. The opinion-shaping potential of television broadcasts lies in repetition. However, it requires a television and (a) viewer(s) that were aplenty during the global lockdowns practiced during 2020. Airways are, however, buzzing with ringtones and notifications in our hands and pockets. Social media also achieves its objectives through repetitions, but unlike regulated broadcast content that drives various commercial entities to compete, it's largely unregulated. Pandemic-related fake news has been widely peddled all along and probably have achieved their objectives of sowing confusion and panic. In fact, public ends up not just the consumer but also the source of unknowingly spreading such information to the utter dismay of television programmers and mass communication gurus. Before various actors and/or stakeholders of this health communication continuum are discussed individually, it's certain that COVID-19 has diversified the health communication pathways. More than ever before, the onus is on the consumer of health information to make informed choices. The era beyond COVID-19 might be "self-regulation." Nevertheless, it adds to the responsibilities of health educators and clinicians to improve not just the quality of their messaging but also the promptness to keep masses and patients self-sufficient and aware of unforeseen medical/public health scenarios.

7.3 Infodemic

Is too much knowledge as dangerous as little knowledge? Ways to differentiate real science from non-science or junk-science must be found. The answer may lie in multi-disciplinary solutions that develop models and platforms inherently capable of picking up authentic information. However, it's substantially resource intensive. On the other hand, available media platforms diverge in their ability and inability to promote what works in COVID pandemic or what does not work. From herbal remedies to faith-based healing, an array of treatment opinions exists bordering on miraculous to conspiratorial origins. The reliability of a particular broadcast/print media is probably being judges by its viewers/readers if the medical journals are to be the yardstick of authenticity of knowledge. Afterall, the number of unreliable journals has long outnumbered the household names that public and health professionals have relied in past few centuries. Despite it, the last 2 years have witnessed unprecedented rate of information flowing between laboratories, researchers, pharmaceutical industry, clinicians, public health specialists, and public. It offers a quantifiable digital and/or scientific footprint invaluable to researchers to inform pandemic preparedness and test various models for authentic information sharing among key actors interconnected in Fig. 7.1. Concurrently, the misleading or irresponsible use of social media during health emergencies (as already witnessed during COVID-19) is a constant challenge to the growth of "informed citizenry."

7.4 Digital Healthcare Models

Strict lockdowns imposed by countries in the last months have contributed to define new interesting ways of health communication between patient-physician and also between all healthcare figures involved in this pandemic.

Thus, in the era of digital health technologies, the focus on new models has shifted to:

- Telehealth for virtual care, virtual visits, and interdisciplinary management.
- Mobile apps for remote patient monitoring.
- Websites and chatbots for risk assessment, screening, triage.

To decrease the risk of infection, telemedicine has been used as a successful healthcare model in both emergency and primary care, including for communications purposes among scientists, clinicians, institutional figures. Moreover, official communication plans should promote facile and diverse channels to inform people about the pandemic and to avoid rumors and reduce threats to public health. Social media platforms are highly beneficial to model pandemic trends as well as to monitor the evolution of patients' symptoms or public reaction to the pandemic over time. However, acceptability and, even concrete availability, of digital solutions may face challenges due to potential conflicts with users' cultural, moral, religious backgrounds, and different socioeconomic scenarios. Overall, digital tools seem provide collective public health benefits; however, they may be considered intrusive and can interfere with individual principles or leave vulnerable-disadvantage populations behind.

7.5 Digital Communication

Good communication strategies help manage people's fear and increase the likelihood that they will adhere to the measures suggested or imposed on them during the crisis. The pandemic has disrupted traditional ways of scientific communication. Communication in epidemics must be clear and unambiguous and also reach the target population quickly (health workers, authorities, and global population). Digital methods appear to be promising solutions, as they enable people to maintain physical distance while keeping informed or maintaining contact with others. Since the beginning of the COVID-19 pandemic, disinformation, "fake news," and conspiracy theories about the origin, spread, and treatment of the disease have been present on the internet and in government communications and social media.

These communication problems also cause confusion and mistrust; the consequences are negative at both the individual and community levels. To provide the most useful information in a timely fashion, effective digital risk communication has been established internationally by WHO as well as nationally and regionally through an active factual information campaign using several digital authoritative channels [5, 6]. The digital formats are decentralized and attract large numbers of viewers from across the globe per lecture, creating a continuous, slow-motion, worldwide conference. Could we do without in-person events entirely? Many would argue "no." Intuition and experience tell us that digital communication and in-person differs dramatically. Both these ways of communication are and will be part of our life and probably influenced by the continuous flow of the events.

7.6 Research Ecosystem During COVID-19 Pandemic

COVID-19 pandemic has imposed a great revolution in the context of the research ecosystem forming new scientific coalitions in record time, opening of new calls across different research groups, the organization of virtual scientific conferences for comparing data and crisis updates, and the launch of a new portal in support of cocreation processes and open science. Moreover, several teleconferences involving various disciplines at the national and international level have taken place. All these efforts provide multiple venues to support the common effort of combating the COVID-19 pandemic. The sharing of evidence-based knowledge and scientific progress is an effective and essential make a difference in this crisis [7]. The abrupt transition to all-digital formats of scientific conferences during the last year may have a positive key of lecture, if considered as a method to promote and in some ways democratize scientific information spread and facilitate professional interdisciplinary and multicenter networking [8]. Although in a cruel manner, the current pandemic has presented an opportunity to adopt new ways to communicate science and build scientific relationships within a digital environment, thereby reducing the environmental impact and increasing the inclusivity of scientific events.

In Table 7.1, we describe the main features (advantages versus disadvantages) of the current digital health and research system in the COVID-19 era, characterized by interesting and complex connections.

Table 7.1 Main features of current digital health and research systems in COVID 19 era

Healthcare system	Advantages	Disadvantages
	• Virtual hospital, virtual care • Telemedicine • e-prescribing • Remote patient monitoring system • Website, chatbot for risk assessment, triage, screening	• Depersonalization of relation patient-physician?
Research and health tech	• Digital formats consents not stop research and teaching programs and respect lockdown restrictions • Digital communication consents multicenters communication by promotion of interaction between researchers across disciplines and countries • Digital cohort studies • Creation of effective epidemiological registrars, platforms • Data sharing • Monitoring online activities and data for incidence prediction, disease spreading models • Promotion of international researcher scholarship programs • Democratization of scientific knowledge spread: going over geographic and financial barriers • Recording of scientific events • Reduction in venue, travel, organizational costs • Environment advantages?	• No in-person events • Non-verbal communication
Population	• Outbreak communication risks: avoid misinformation, fake news, conspiracy theories • Smartphone-based tracking, interactive web-based dashboard • Use of official digital communication strategies	• Concerns about privacy?

7.7 Post-Crisis Communication: The Long View

Communication during a crisis is always a challenge and even more so with the unprecedented COVID-19 pandemic. In a cruel manner, this pandemic may contribute to discover and improve new ways to do research and clinical practice and to communicate each other everywhere. Pandemic has revealed the strong potential of various digital health solutions that have been tested during the last months. Obviously, more concerted measures should be implemented to ensure that future digital health initiatives will be improved and have a greater impact on the epidemic and meet the most strategic needs to face the crisis and may leave useful tools in eredity for the future of research and clinical approaches.

The COVID-19 pandemic may be a reminder that besides our duty to care, we are committed to improve. By meeting these challenges today, we may be able to enrich scientific research and provide better care to future patients [6, 9–11]. Experts described how virtual conferences are more inclusive, more affordable, less time-consuming, and more accessible worldwide, especially for early-career researchers. Making conferences more open and inclusive will provide both immediate and long-term benefits to the scientific community [12]. A culture of open digital communication, group reviews, and live national and international discussions will strengthen scientific bonds among researchers in all disciplines.

Are online science events, digital healthcare system here to stay? In a recent Nature reader poll, more than 80% of respondents said that they would be in favor of some scientific conferences remaining virtual after the COVID-19 era [13]. We want to conclude with some questions? [1] Has COVID-19 served as a catalyst for already-brewing attempts to review and modernize the methods of clinical and scientific discourse? [2] When the pandemic is tamed and normality becomes possible again, should we return to our old ways? Probably no … This pandemic is re-designing scenarios in each field of life. Communication is evidently the tool that can address the two tracks this pandemic has created for those who can afford the available treatments and vaccines and those who cannot.

References

1. Mahmood S, Hasan K, Colder Carras M, Labrique A. Global preparedness against COVID-19: we must leverage the power of digital health. JMIR Public Health Surveill. 2020;6(2):e18980. https://doi.org/10.2196/18980.
2. Center for Systems Science and Engineering at Johns Hopkins University. 2020. COVID-19 Dashboard https://coronavirus.jhu.edu/map.html.
3. Reeves JJ, Hollandsworth HM, Torriani FJ, Taplitz R, Abeles S, Tai-Seale M, Millen M, Clay BJ, Longhurst CA. Rapid response to COVID-19: health informatics support for outbreak management in an academic health system. J Am Med Inform Assoc. 2020;27(6):853–9. https://doi.org/10.1093/jamia/ocaa037.
4. Power B. The Washington Post, 2020. Mar 27 [2020-04-21]. The coronavirus is expanding the surveillance state. How will this play out? https://www.washingtonpost.com/politics/2020/03/27/coronavirus-is-expanding-surveillance-state-how-will-this-play-out/.

5. Fagherazzi G, Goetzinger C, Rashid MA, Aguayo GA, Huiart L. Digital health strategies to fight COVID-19 worldwide: challenges, recommendations, and a call for papers. J Med Internet Res. 2020;22(6):e19284.
6. Arabi YM, Azoulay E, Al-Dorzi HM, Phua J, Salluh J, Binnie A, et al. How the COVID-19 pandemic will change the future of critical care. Intensive Care Med. 2021;47(3):282–91.
7. Mandal H. Mobilizing the research ecosystem for scientific advances towards positive impact in the context of the COVID-19 pandemic. Turk J Med Sci. 2020;50:485–8.
8. Banerjee R, Kelkar AH, Logan AC, Majhail NS, Pemmaraju N. The democratization of scientific conferences: twitter in the era of COVID-19 and beyond. Curr Hematol Malig Rep. 2021;16:1–8. https://doi.org/10.1007/s11899-021-00620-w.
9. Bottanelli F, Cadot B, Campelo F, Curran S, Davidson PM, Dey G, et al. Science during lockdown – from virtual seminars to sustainable online communities. J Cell Sci. 2020;133(15):jcs249607.
10. Viglione GA. Year without conferences? How the coronavirus pandemic could change research. Nature. 2020;579(7799):327–8. https://doi.org/10.1038/d41586-020-00786-y.
11. Bozelos PA, Vogels TP. Talking science, online. Nat Rev Neurosci. 2020;22:1–2. https://doi.org/10.1038/s41583-020-00408-6.
12. Sarabipour S. Virtual conferences raise standards for accessibility and interactions. Elife. 2020;9:e62668.
13. Coronavirus in charts: the fact-checkers correcting falsehoods. Nature. 2020.

Chapter 8
The "Traditional" Meetings and Congresses

Jonathan P. Wyatt

8.1 The Background to Medical Meetings

Medical practitioners and academics have held meetings in a formalised way to share practice and ideas for a long time. The Medical and Chirurgical Society of London held meetings as long ago as 1805, subsequently becoming the Royal Society of Medicine and expanding their range of meetings to the current day [1]. During the twentieth century, medical conferences became an integral part of the way that new ideas in medicine were presented, discussed, and developed. It became standard for most branches of medicine and their respective colleges and societies to hold regular conferences and meetings to bring like-minded members together in a spirit of shared learning and exploration. A variety of terms are used (often interchangeably) to describe these medical meetings (Table 8.1)—the term "conference" is perhaps the best default. Courses are part of an altogether different category, usually following a rigid structure and incorporating specific outcomes.

8.2 The Reasons for Meetings

The principal reason that underpins many medical conferences and meetings is to share and exchange ideas and results within the general aim of advancing healthcare. Presentations of original research are at the core of medical meetings and conferences. Researchers use them as a means of first presenting their findings to the world and opening up their methods, results, and conclusions to the scrutiny of

J. P. Wyatt (✉)
University of Exeter Medical School, Exeter, UK
e-mail: jpwyatt@nhs.net

G. C. Di Renzo (ed.), *Essential Writing, Communication and Narrative Skills for Medical Scientists Before and After the COVID Era*,
https://doi.org/10.1007/978-3-030-84954-2_8

Table 8.1 Medical meeting types and terminology

Term	Implication/meaning
Conference	Standard term used to describe a formalised event, bringing together individuals with a shared interest, often lasting for several days and involving hundreds of attendees
Congress	Typically used to describe a large international conference. Implies that those attending (delegates) are members of a regulatory organisation that issues rules and guidance
Convention	Also sometimes used to describe a large meeting, which may have a political element in terms of decision-making about practices at work
Course	A specific type of meeting, quite separate from a conference, in which attendees learn about a particular topic, according to a rigid structure
Meeting	General umbrella term which covers the whole range of small gatherings and larger events
Symposium	A focused meeting to explore a particular topic (as opposed to the broad range of topics at a conference), usually only lasting for a day or less
Webinar	Online presentation and/or interaction involving one or more speakers and an audience
Workshop	Often an element of a larger meeting/conference in which individuals explore a particular subject in detail with one or more experts

peers and other experts. The discussion of original research enables related ideas to be developed. In addition to engaging in formal presentations and discussion, researchers also use the conference setting as an opportunity to informally network with like-minded individuals and potential collaborators in future research. This collaboration may occur within the confines of the conference halls or outside this in the more informal settings, such as bars and restaurants.

Most of the individuals who attend medical meetings and conferences are probably not motivated by a desire to share their original research findings, ideas, or knowledge, but want to improve their learning and understanding of subjects relevant to their work. Formalised meetings enable attendees the chance to update their understanding and knowledge of relevant specialist areas and to learn/practice skills. In addition, attendance also enables individuals to meet continuing professional development (CPD) requirements, both for their immediate employer and for the relevant specialty governing body (e.g. colleges). Conferences offer opportunities for all attendees to catch up with previous colleagues and engage in "networking," which includes a variety of activities, ranging from collaboration in projects to applying for jobs. For many, attending a conference allows those attending to escape from some of the usual work pressures and provides an opportunity to focus and learn without distraction. Many conferences offer a social programme to accompany the academic one, which can be highly prized by those attending.

Over the past 40 years, numerous medical courses have been established, often by colleges and regulatory organisations, with the aim of training up medical professionals in a particular area and have become very popular. One of the earliest was the Advanced Trauma Life Support course, set up by the American College of Surgeons in 1977 [2]. Although the courses have some similarities in structure with medical conferences, the focus is quite different, in that rather than exploring the boundaries of current theory and practice, the courses teach in an efficient and didactic manner to achieve specific levels of knowledge and competence.

8.3 Choice of Venue

The venues selected to host events include hotels, purpose built conference centres, universities, and colleges. Some colleges and large organisations that run annual or regular meetings have a policy of rotating venues around a number of countries and/or cities according to predetermined agreement. Conference organisers who are responsible for choosing a venue need to consider of a number of (sometimes competing) factors, including the following:

- A city/location which will be both accessible and attractive to a large number and range of potential attendees.
- Adequate space/number of rooms, including areas for commercial stands.
- Optimal educational environment.
- Minimum audio-visual presentation and Wi-Fi requirements.
- Nearby accommodation and planned social activities.
- Cost of hiring the venue.

8.3.1 Classical Conference Structure

Most large conferences follow a traditional structure which has been well described [3]. Meetings are usually opened and closed with an address to all those attending. Lectures delivered to all attendees ("plenary sessions") may be used to open (and close) meetings. This includes a "keynote address" in which an eminent individual sets the tone and establishes the themes for the conference or summarises proceedings at the end. In addition to running sessions for all attendees, larger meetings typically run several tracks at the same time, whereby those attending can choose which sessions they wish to attend. These "breakout" sessions include lectures, seminars, research presentations, discussion groups, workshops, and skills sessions. Sometimes, these breakout sessions need to be booked up or reserved in advance by attendees—space constraints inherent in the venue may limit the number that can attend each session.

The core feature that underpins academic meetings is the presentation of original research. The standard format is for researchers to present a summary of their projects in presentations lasting for 20–30 min to include some time for discussion and questions from the audience. Technological advances have changed the way that this occurs (see below), but the process encourages a significant degree of academic scrutiny to be applied and for researchers in a particular field to explore ideas together. For many meetings, getting a paper accepted for oral presentation is a competitive process and becomes a line on the researcher's curriculum vitae. In addition, many prestigious meetings publish the summaries of the research presentations as conference proceedings or abstracts in relevant journals, often with these available as a printed (and/or electronic) handout at the meeting. The publication of abstracts in scientific medical journals has traditionally acted as a way for medical researchers to get relevant early attention for their work.

For those researchers whose work does not quite meet the standard of being presented orally, most conferences provide opportunities for poster presentations, whereby posters are displayed in a hall for delegates to read, together with some formalised sessions in which the presenters can add a short oral presentation and answer questions, often as part of a moderated multiple track session, with a prize awarded to the best poster.

In addition to oral research presentations and poster presentations, the twin or multiple track format of many conferences also comprises breakout sessions of seminars, discussion groups, and workshops. These usually have a focused aim which may be relevant to the theme of the conference. Seminars are based on experts discussing and sharing ideas and information, whereas practical workshops focus on delegates learning and practising skills—occasionally, these are arranged in a separate event prior to or following the main conference.

Some conferences are arranged by colleges and large specialty organisations. An integral part of some of these meetings are annual general and other meetings, which help to determine the direction of the organisation. These may include voting for formal roles and the presentation of awards following examinations.

Conferences enable opportunities for "section meetings" of subspecialty interest groups and various other groups related to the overall theme. These include meetings of journal editorial committees, examiner groups, trainees' groups, and guideline writers. Rather than being embedded within it, some of these meetings use the conference as an opportunity to get relevant individuals together outside of the formal conference setting.

Commercial organisations help to reduce costs of large conferences by sponsorship and paying to display their wares at stalls within the halls, typically targeting coffee and lunch breaks. Organisations potentially interested in having a stall include book sellers, equipment manufacturers, smaller/sister organisations, and organisers of exam revision courses.

The classical conference structure incorporates some social events, at which individuals are able to network and share ideas with like-minded colleagues from different areas. Social events may be formalised into grand dinners or be more informal, incorporating visits to local places of interest, either of an academic or sometimes purely tourist nature. Venues in exotic places may also encourage individuals to attend by offering a social programme which may include sporting trips. This might support the feeling that attending a conference should feel a bit special and act as a reward for working hard all year. Finally, the role of informal networking aspect of medical meetings should not be underestimated. Conferences are used as an opportunity to approach individuals about jobs and involvement in other academic projects.

8.4 Evolution of Conference Technology over Time

The experience of attending medical meetings has changed considerably over time, as advances in technology transformed the way that ideas and information are delivered, shared, and discussed. Overhead projectors were in widespread use in all fields of education during the latter half of the twentieth century [4] but were largely replaced by slide projectors at medical meetings. These allowed a carousel of 35 mm colour slides to be projected on a screen, with areas of interest on individual slides to be identified by the presenter by using a laser pointer. Despite the efforts of projectionists hired by conferences to manage the slide projectors, presentations could be troubled by numerous issues: lack of focus, slides inserted (and then projected) the wrong way round and upside down, slides jamming in the machine, and even melting [5]. Technological advances in computers at the end of the twentieth century resulted in the widespread adoption of Microsoft's PowerPoint for electronic presentations at medical and other meetings [6]. These presentations have developed to be able to incorporate videos and other media, but are not immune from (Information Technology) issues whereby the presentation fails to load and/or play properly.

Technology has also impacted the way that a presenter can interact with the audience. During presentations, the presenter can ask the audience to "vote" electronically and display the results immediately to enable further discussion. Similarly, rather than take questions at the end of a presentation in an unprepared fashion, the person chairing the session can receive questions and comments electronically (e.g. via Twitter) and put them to the presenter without the need for a roaming microphone—something which might appeal to more shy members of the audience. Conference organisers can also use social media (e.g. Twitter, Facebook) to interact with attendees, including providing updates relating to both the academic and social aspects of the programme of the meeting.

The presentation of posters is a well-established part of many medical conferences. These were originally physically cumbersome, as either large boards with paper pasted on, or in the form of large scrolls. Posters are now typically produced and submitted in electronic form and can be the focus of attention at the meeting by being projected onto physical screens and/or made available for viewing electronically.

8.5 Problems with Conferences

Medical meetings and conferences are associated with some issues, which are summarised in Table 8.2. Depending exactly which city is going to host a meeting and where the attendees will be coming from, a considerable amount of travel may be necessary, incurring financial and travel costs, which require to be covered by those attending and their employing institutions. Large international

Table 8.2 Problems with traditional conferences

Area of issue	Problems
Access-related	• Cost and time of travel to venue • Safety and security • Carbon footprint of travel
Venue-related	• Cost of hiring • Size and number of rooms required • Access to accommodation • Information technology issues • Catering issues
Attender-related	• Cost • Time away from caring responsibilities • Difficult to get time off work • Large impersonal feel • Lack of comfort • Inability to see from the back of a hall • Risk of acquiring infection

conferences have been criticised because of the carbon footprint of those travelling to get there [7]. In addition, there may limitations of travel access to certain cities.

Finding the perfect venue within a city can prove to be quite a challenge for organisers. This is particularly true for larger events, for which the choice of venues capable of hosting large numbers of attendees is likely to be limited. Even once a potential venue has been identified and is available, there are other important considerations. These include hiring costs, safety and security issues, availability of reliable wireless networking (Wi-Fi) and related information technology systems, catering support, and access to accommodation.

Attending a medical meeting at some distance from home is not without issues. Some researchers, scientists, practitioners, and students (especially at the start of their careers) may not manage to secure funding to attend. Apart from the costs involved, travel time to and from the venue is also a consideration, particularly for those with caring responsibilities at home, who may find it difficult to get cover for the time that they are away. Some of those attending a conference may struggle to see and hear the presentations from the back of a crowded hall, whilst others may find a large conference to be a slightly impersonal affair. Even without these issues, most attendees are likely to return home tired after a busy conference and long journey, yet whilst having been away for a few days, the expectations of work and family are likely to be that they should throw themselves straight back into their regular respective roles at work and at home.

Finally, from 2020 onwards, there is the new possibility of acquiring COVID-19 whilst away. The new disease has changed the way that medical scientists and professionals have approached attending conferences. However, the association between conferences and infectious diseases is nothing new: in 1976, more than a hundred Legionnaires attending a national three-day convention in Philadelphia became ill and many died of an acute respiratory infection [8].

8.6 The Effect of COVID-19 on Conferences

At the end of 2019 and during the first few months on 2020, the coronavirus (SARS-Cov-2) responsible for COVID-19 spread from Wuhan, China, around the world, resulting in a pandemic. The disease stretched medical care to the limit in regions of several countries, including China and Italy, with large numbers of patients requiring oxygen and ventilator support. Initial reports were that it spread by close contact, especially involving respiratory droplets, and that it carried an overall estimated mortality rate of approximately 2% [9]. It was also apparent that infected individuals could spread the disease whilst still asymptomatic. Given this background, it is no surprise that gatherings of large numbers of individuals at meetings and conferences, resulted in spread of the disease. A multinational biotechnology company held a "leadership conference" in Boston, USA, in late February 2020 involving 175 individuals from around the world, and within days, there were 70 coronavirus infections linked to the meeting [10]. This medical conference quickly became famous as being a "superspreading" event. Soon after, several large organisations cancelled or postponed their annual conferences: this included the Royal College of Physicians in the UK and the American College of Physicians in the USA [11]. Numerous healthcare conferences around the world were cancelled as the pandemic spread and whole countries instigated "lockdown" measures [12].

Concern has been expressed in the academic world that cancellation of conferences could have a negative effect on the overall advancement of scientific research [13]. These cancellations have a number of potential implications for the research community in a number of ways:

- Inability of research findings to be presented and discussed.
- Abstracts/conference proceedings not getting published.
- Difficulties for researchers to network and form plans for future work.
- Delay of career progression of researchers and academics.
- Costs incurred by learned societies of cancelling meetings.

8.7 COVID-19 and Research

Just at the moment when the medical research community was being severely affected by the COVID-19 pandemic, the world needed it to function most effectively in order to provide the answers as to how to combat the disease. Considering the rapidity with which the disease was spreading, it became quickly clear that solutions in terms of both treatments and vaccines were required much more quickly than allowed by the usual research process and publication.

The concept of rapid pre-publication data release in medical science is not new [14], but was put under the spotlight by COVID-19 with hundreds of organisations agreeing to share research data from January 2020 onwards [15, 16]. The fast-track process and release of results of studies on possible drugs to treat COVID-19 has been unusual and perplexing. First, disappointing data from a Chinese study on the antiviral agent remdesivir was leaked and posted on the World Health Organization website, before being withdrawn; and then less than a week later, the director of the US National Institute of Allergy and Infectious Diseases revealed its positive effect on recovery in a press conference at the White House [17, 18]. There followed the retraction of a paper on the efficacy of hydroxychloroquine/chloroquine in the Lancet which caused some confusion [19, 20]. The first study demonstrating a mortality reduction from a drug released its results on use of dexamethasone in a press conference, although it was greeted cautiously in some quarters (as "science by press release"), which was perhaps not surprising, considering what had gone before with other drugs [21].

Despite these well-publicised issues surrounding the studies on managing COVID-19, there has been remarkable cooperation between healthcare workers and researchers around the world in sharing best practice via the internet. At the end of March 2020, more than 130,000 viewers from 160 countries participated in the European Society of Intensive Care Medicine's COVID Marathon webinar [22]. The way that so many individuals were able and willing to adapt to use new technologies is quite impressive.

8.8 The Shift to Online Meeting and Working

Workers around the world in a wide range of occupations have quickly shifted to working at home during the COVID-19 crisis. Unsurprisingly, remote working was embraced early by large technology companies, including Facebook, Square, and Twitter [23]. Medical practitioners have adapted quickly in the workplace, both in terms of patient—clinician interactions and clinician—clinician/management interactions. Academics within the fields of medicine and medical science have also moved quickly to provide teaching, meetings, supervision, and even examinations online, using technology (e.g. Microsoft Teams, Zoom) which has become familiar within many homes [24]. Employees are gradually getting used to this technology and how to use it to make the most from working from home [25]. Whilst some advantages are obvious (no travel to work time/cost, no risk of acquiring infectious disease), others can have a downside (it is good for employees not to have to worry about arranging childcare, but children can also prove to be a significant distraction during work time).

8.9 The Future of Conferences and Medical Meetings

The need for medical academics, professionals, and scientists to meet is clear, but it is equally clear that the traditional format of meetings and conferences is not feasible in the short-term without making dramatic changes, whilst the risk of COVID-19 remains. It might be possible to mitigate some risks to try to run a conference in a traditional style (e.g. by temperature screening attendees on arrival, introducing social distancing measures or by running hybrid meetings, comprising a mixture of in-person meetings with on-line attendances [26]). However, it seems more likely that in the medium term, current trends will continue in terms of a significant shift to online conferences and Webinars, which may become embedded as researchers and academics rethink the way that they interact [27].

8.10 Conferences as Virtual Events

Some medical meetings and conferences which were planned to be held as meeting in person events have already been transformed into virtual events [28]. Widespread availability of internet access means that attendees can join meetings from their offices and homes.

Lectures and presentations (including research presented as part of free paper sessions) can all be relatively easily distributed using online technology. Webinars (online live interactive sessions incorporating or permitting discussion, polls and surveys) facilitate involvement and interaction. Technology allows sessions to be recorded and viewed later. Webinars enable a session to be followed up by material being added later to cover questions asked and to clarify issues that require additional attention. Numerous options are available which can be chosen to be the delivery platform for webinars. Potential advantages from a personal point of view of attendees watching a presentation from home or office rather than in a lecture hall are that they can:

- Sit comfortably in informal attire.
- Watch with a clear view, without heads obstructing.
- Hear clearly.
- Choose exactly when to watch and when not to watch (without having to walk out of a crowded auditorium).
- Record and watch later, including tracks occurring simultaneously.

Many workshops are amenable to being done online in an interactive fashion. However, this might be more tricky when the focus is on learning or perfecting some practical skills, although arguably equipment could be prepared/spread in advance, as occurs with online surgical training.

Posters and poster presentation sessions can be easily managed online. Similarly, sponsors and/or advertisers can still play a part in virtual conferences. Messages and adverts can be displayed on banners and appear in the programme notes.

Social interaction and networking are recognised to be important for researchers and are key elements of a conference [29]. It is hard to find an immediate way to replace a formal conference dinner and the networking that accompanies it. However, if the world of digital dating post-COVID-19 is anything to go by, then there may be more potential to make progress in this respect than is immediately

Table 8.3 Summary of the advantages of holding virtual conferences

Perspective	Advantage
Attendee	• Reduced costs • Ease of booking/logging in • Reduced travel time • More flexible experience • Attendees can get what they want from it • No risk of COVID-19 or other infections
Host	• Reduced cost • Unlimited numbers of attendees • Reduced venue-related issues
Other	• Reduced carbon footprint

apparent [30]. Furthermore, even before COVID-19, scientists were already well versed with social networking—there is no reason why conference organisers cannot innovate and harness social networks to their advantage and that of their attendees [31].

8.11 The Benefits of Holding a Virtual Conference

The advantages of holding a conference virtually are summarised in Table 8.3. From the perspective of those attending, the costs of attending the conference, travelling to get there, and staying there are obviously much reduced. There are similar advantages when it comes to saving time, especially in relation to travelling to and from the venue, so that delegates may return to work after the conference relatively fresh rather than "jet-lagged." Online attendance offers delegates the potential for a more informal, flexible experience, with no risk of acquiring COVID-19 from delegates sitting next to them. The flexibility may include sorting out carer responsibilities and watching some presentations later.

From the perspective of the host, organising an online conference does not carry with it the restrictions of finding a venue which is physically big enough. Similarly, issues of catering and accommodation at the venue are also removed. The cost of holding a conference is also reduced. Environmentally aware individuals will consider it to be important that the carbon footprint of an online conference is obviously also significantly reduced.

8.12 Potential Disadvantages of Holding a Virtual Conference

The potential disadvantages of holding a conference virtually rather than in person are summarised in Table 8.4. Attending a conference from home may be convenient, but may feel more impersonal and not quite so special as travelling to a

Table 8.4 Summary of problems with virtual conferences

Perspective	Disadvantage
Attendee	• Requires functioning Wi-fi/internet • Zoom fatigue • Impersonal and not very engaging • External distractions (family, work) • Hard to replicate social interaction/networking • Hard to replicate the experience of visiting a new place
Host	• Technology can still fail • Hard to replicate some elements at home
Other	• Colleges/organisations lose income stream

distant venue. Successful engagement in a meeting does require a functioning internet connection and a quiet space free from external distractions (e.g. work colleagues or family members demanding attention). Linking and interacting with a conference by video conferencing can be quite tiring and detract from the overall experience being offered. A number of reasons have been put forward as explanations for what is sometimes referred to as "Zoom fatigue," with commentators advising regular breaks between sessions to minimise it—something which virtual conference organisers may want to consider [32, 33]. It is very difficult for a virtual conference to replicate the cultural experience that is involved in visiting a new place, but it is possible for an online conference to run with a cultural theme, in addition to an academic one. The challenge of recreating the social experience and networking that is an invariable part of attending a conference has already been described above.

Online conferences might spare organisers from having concerns about physical space constraints relating to a venue, but issues about technology failure remain. It is likely that additional funding will need to be spent on supporting technological solutions and emergency support in the event of problems. Issues about funding are relevant in other respects: many Colleges and leaned societies use income from conferences and meetings as an important income stream—at first thought, it may be hard to justify a large attendance fee for an online event.

8.13 The Hybrid Conference

Holding a meeting both in person and available to attend on line arguably offers the best of both worlds. This "hybrid conference" would enable the delegate the option which would best suit their personal circumstances. So for example, the potential attendee with health issues (e.g. immunosuppressed) and concerns about travelling or who cannot secure time and/or funding to attend (e.g. student) could attend virtually (at a reduced cost). At the other extreme, the researcher keen to meet in person and engage fully in the cultural experience and social/networking programme would be able to attend in person.

8.14 Conclusions

COVID-19 has affected a lot of things that had become a part of everyday life. Some things will never be the same again—old-fashioned, traditional conferences may be amongst these. Many individuals, including in the academic and scientific community, have adapted and become accustomed to new ways of living and working—some are thinking afresh about their priorities and lifestyle. The need for medical scientists, academics, researchers, and practitioners to meet and share ideas, research, and practice is greater than ever in the post-COVID era. Technology can offer solutions which enable most of the functions of physical face-to-face meetings to be replaced (or duplicated) online, and whilst there are challenges in some areas, the benefits in others should be acknowledged and embraced.

References

1. Hunting P. The royal society of medicine. Postgrad Med J. 2005;81(951):45–8.
2. Carmont MR. The advanced trauma life support course: a history of its development and review of related literature. Postgrad Med J. 2005;81:87–91.
3. Wyatt J. Organising a medical conference. J Accid Emerg Med. 1999;16:223–6.
4. 3M. A century of innovation: the 3M story. St.Paul: 3M; 2002.
5. Ward CW, Wilkinson AE. Conducting meaningful interpretation: a field guide for success. Golden: Fulcrum Publishing; 2006.
6. Davies R. 29 reasons to love PowerPoint. https://www.wired.co.uk/article/powerpoint-brithday-defence. New York: Wired UK Conde Nast Publications; 2016.
7. Grémillet D. Paradox of flying to meetings to protect the environment. Nature. 2008;455:1175.
8. Edelstein PH, Roy CR. Legionnaires' disease and Pontiac fever. In: Mandell, Douglas, and Bennetts principles and practice of infectious diseases. 8th ed; 2015.
9. Wyatt JP, Taylor RG, Hotton E, de Wit K. Oxford handbook of emergency medicine. 5th ed. Oxford: Oxford University Press; 2020.
10. Arsenault M. How the Biogen leadership conference in Boston spread the coronavirus. *The Boston Globe*, 10th March 2020.
11. Rimmer A. Covid-19: Medical conferences around the world are cancelled after US cases are linked to Massachusetts meeting. BMJ. 2020;368:1054.
12. Robbins R. STAT's guide to health care conferences disrupted by the coronavirus crisis. https://www.statnews.com/2020/03/07stats-guide-health-care-conferences-disrupted-covid-19/.
13. Bothwell E. Conference cancellations could have "big impact" on research. *Times Higher Education*. 11th March 2020.
14. Toronto 2009 Data Release Workshop Authors. Benefits and best practices of rapid pre-publication data release. Nature. 2009;461(7261):168–70.
15. Academy of Medical Royal Colleges. Sharing research data and findings relevant to the novel coronavirus (COVID-19) outbreak. Wellcome Trust. https://wellcome.ac.uk/coronavirus-covid-19/open-data.
16. Moorthy V, Restrepo AMH, Preziosi M-P, Swaminathan S. Data sharing for novel coronavirus (COVID-19). Bull World Health Organ. 2020;98:150.
17. Park A. Leaked data from a key remdesivir study suggest the potential coronavirus drug is not effective. *Time*. 23 April 2020. https://time.com/5826618/remdesivir-leaked-data-who-website/.

18. Kuchler H, Mancini DP. Fauci praises remdesivir after data show it speeds recovery. *Financial Times*. 29 April 2020. https://www.ft.com/content/1625275b-9981-49f4-b788-661f8243890d/.
19. Mehra MR, Ruschitzka F, Patel AN. Retraction-Hydroxychloroquine or chloroquine with or without a macrolide for treatment of COVID-19: a multinational registry analysis. Lancet. 2020;195:1820. https://doi.org/10.1016/S0140-6736(20)31324-6/.
20. Boseley S, Davey M. Covid-19: Lancet retracts paper that halted hydroxychloroquine trials. Guardian. 2020; https://www.theguardian.com/world/2020/jun/04/covid-19-lancet-retracts-paper-that-halted-hydroxychloroquine-trials/
21. Ledford H. Coronavirus breakthrough: dexamethasone is first drug shown to save lives. Nature 2020;582:469.
22. European Society of Intensive Care Intensivists Care for Lives! Connect and share with ICU professionals facing COVID-19! 2020. https://esicm-tv.org/covid19.
23. Murphy H. Facebook to shift permanently to a more remote workforce. *Financial Times*. 21 May 2020. https://www.ft.com/content/4ae2fdf7-f427-4e98-abd7-feeb6b6f43f2.
24. Mukherjee S, Rana A. Zoom takes lead over Microsoft Teams as virus keeps Americans at home: apptopia. *Reuters: Technology News*, 31 March 2020.
25. Weed J. How to succeed in your office job when there is no office. *The New York Times*. 22 June 2020. https://www.nytimes.com/2020/06/21/business/work-home-coronavirus.html.
26. Lanz LH. Boston hospitality review. What will conferences look like post-COVID-19. 2020. https://www.bu.edu/bhr/2020/04/16/what-will-conferences-look-like-post-covid-19/.
27. Viglione G. A year without conferences? How the coronavirus pandemic could change research. Nature. 2020;579:327.
28. European Society of Radiology. Medical conferences in the post-COVID world: a challenge, and an opportunity. Eur Radiol. 2020;30:5533. https://doi.org/10.1007/s00330-020-06933-3.
29. Gotian R. Networking for introverted scientists. Nature. 2019; http://www.nature.com/articles/d41586-019-01296-2
30. Darbyshire M. Digital dating: why my love life is flourishing under lockdown. *Financial Times*. 16 April 2020. https://www.ft.com/content/5eedb876-7e6a-11ea-82f6-150830b3b99a.
31. Van Noorden R. Online collaboration: Scientists and the social network. Nature. 2014; https://www.nature.com/news/online-collaboration-scientists-and-the-social-network-1.15711
32. Jiang M. The reason Zoom calls drain your energy. *BBC*, 22 Apr 2020. https://www.bbc.com/worklife/article/20200421-why-zoom-video-chats-are-so-exhausting.
33. Walsh K. Zoom fatigue: how to politely decline a call during quarantine. *The New York Times*, 20 May 2020. https://www.nytimes.com/2020/05/20/smarter-living/coronavirus-zoom-facetime-fatigue.html.

Chapter 9
The New Ways to Communicate Your Research: Webinars and Beyond

Alexandre Manuel Henriques Almeida

9.1 Year 2020: The Rise of Webinars

Webinars are an integrant part of our life for some time now, even that we did not refer to them as webinars.

Webinars, also known as web-based seminars, go back in time more than one might initially think. We can lapse into the 1980s with the rise of the internet and the real-time text messaging like IRC (Internet Relay Chat) that was used by individuals and organizations to communicate, share, play and work with each other through IRC networks around the world. In the 1990s, webchats and instant messaging software started to be developed.

These tools were already a kind of webinar even that the term was not yet used as such.

It was in the middle of the 1990s that PictureTel launched the first videoconferencing software and the first public web conferences started to be organised due to the investment of Microsoft on NetMeeting that was incorporated in Internet Explorer web browser. Xerox PARC was the first company to create a software specifically for webinars which already included features like audience polling, private chat communication and the participation of a webinar attendee as a presenter.

From the end of the 1990s and beginning of the 2000s, there was a boom of software for webinars like Webex [2], GoToWebinar [3], ClickWebinar [4] and MyOwnConference [5].

Nowadays, there are dozens of software available that features the most common functionalities of a webinar platform: participant roles, screen, audio and video

A. M. H. Almeida (✉)
Department at Globaz, SA (LOBA), Oliveira de Azeméis, Aveiro, Portugal
e-mail: alexandre@loba.pt

G. C. Di Renzo (ed.), *Essential Writing, Communication and Narrative Skills for Medical Scientists Before and After the COVID Era*,
https://doi.org/10.1007/978-3-030-84954-2_9

sharing, registration and invitation management, chat and Q&A, file transfer, raise hand, pooling, live stream to social media and dial from phones.

With the unfortunate event of COVID-19, the webinars took a special role for the organisation of events and also in the communication of science and research results. All around the globe we saw how physical events where first cancelled or postponed and then, when the situation worsened, events where substituted for webinars, with the necessary restructuration. Thus, it is now of paramount importance that researchers and scientists use these high-level tools for research communication with peers and other stakeholders (policy-makers, investors, partners, society, etc.).

9.2 What Can a Webinar Do for Research and Science Communication?

In the present days, we can consider a webinar to be a vital channel for science communication, especially right now—with COVID-19 forcing so many events and conferences to adapt into a virtual environment. These virtual events are a great way to make audiences feel inspired and ready to act on what has been presented. Moreover, webinars give the opportunity to build a personal relationship and interactions with the audience.

If communication could be seen as a bridge between researchers and the rest of the world, then webinars can be seen as pillar of that bridge, being one of the best tools to guarantee the two-way dialogue that is the baseline of any communication action.

9.3 The Target Audience [6]

When targeting different groups, it is important to use communication strategies best suited to each group. Therefore, the best way to communicate research achievements and insights to different target groups depends on their profiles.

If the objective is to organise a webinar for *general public*, then it is needed to understand that they represent a diverse audience, before being a professor, a researcher, a scientist, a consultant, a housewife, a labourer, an entrepreneur, a policy maker, etc., they are all citizens with their needs, concerns, expectations, families and friends. Using that cape, a citizen is not interested in scientific achievements nor knowledge, they want to know about tangible results and how they impact in the day to day life, they need to know about the real benefits for their life and those around them.

It is also important to take into account the age group of the audience, young people for instance, likes to know to what extent something that is happening in the present will have impact in the future.

When the audience of a webinar are *policy makers*, the focus should be on how science, innovation and quality of life are linked. These group will be interested in understanding the political implications of research results and the impact resulting from the research results achieved. Furthermore, the information provided should be evidence-based, clear and straightforward.

In other hand, if the objective is to communicate to the peers, i.e. other *scientists and researchers* you need to consider that, in principle, this will be the most knowledgeable audience, they will want to know more details about the research than the previous target groups, and, how the research can contribute to the subsequent progress of knowledge, the formation of disciplines and curricula, training, and capacity building.

Finally, if the target group is the *media*, you need to pay attention if the role of the media in the context of your research is to act as an intermediary in communicating results. When approached correctly, the wider world of media is a powerful tool for disseminating knowledge and results to other target groups.

9.4 The Structure of a Webinar

Picking the right webinar format is also important. You have several options and flexibility in the format and style of the webinar, for example, you can use a video studio setup hosted by a single presenter, with a Q&A section for the audience to be involved, or you can follow an interview Q&A-style with two speakers, or a panel discussion with numerous guests and a moderator, or even organise just an audio webinar supported with slides.

Therefore, once you know your audience, the topic that will be covered and the resources available to you, it is important to carefully define the structure and format of the action:

- One expert presenter
- Dual presenters
- E-learning
- Interview
- Panel or roundtable
- Q&A

As mentioned above, defining the structure of a webinar is not a rigid process. It allows mixing different formats to better match with your needs and goals, i.e. you can have a first part with one keynote speaker, followed by a second session with an interview and finish with a Q&A session.

Frequently, interactivity with the audience is crucial for the success of the event, (i.e. collecting feedback, comments and questions); hence whenever possible, the integration of Q&A, chats and raise-hands features should be considered. For this purpose, there are interactive tools, such as the Mentimeter [7] application that allows live quizzes, polls, word clouds, etc. which can ease the interaction and feedback gathering, mainly with larger audiences.

The images below, taken from the webinar [8] organised by LIFT project [9], shows two examples of interactions with the participants: graphic and word cloud (Figs. 9.1 and 9.2).

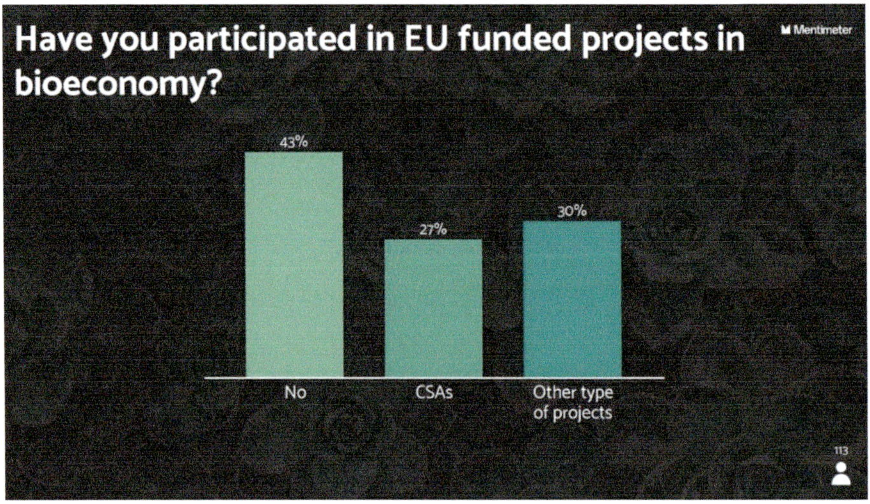

Fig. 9.1 Example [1] of Mentimeter interaction—Graphic

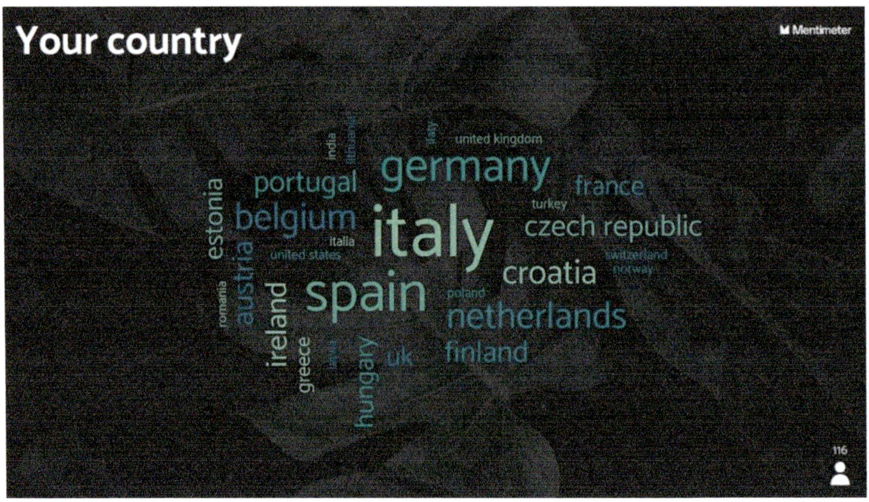

Fig. 9.2 Example [2] of Mentimeter interaction—Word cloud

Keep in mind that webinars are designed to allow two-way communication and audience engagement. This can be done via *chat, Q&A session, running polls and using the raise hand functionality that the common webinar software provides.*

Remember, when people are watching your webinar, they are at their desks in front of a computer, at home or at the office, or they may even be using their mobile device, so they may be tempted to open other websites, check emails or continue with other work while you are speaking.

To keep people engaged, use poll questions, slide decks, and images to keep the attention, and enable your audience to regularly interact. Creative designs can also help to foster better engagement and memory. Embrace simplicity [10].

In terms of duration, according with the analysis made by GoToWebinar [11], 60-min webinars are the most popular. So, try to schedule a 1-h webinar with time at the end for a Q&A session.

From the last years organising webinars, one of the most important feedback that we have received from the participants regards with the added-value of having the speakers always visible on the screen, so… *keep your camera ON*. It makes the experience more personal and engaging for the participants.

In summary when organizing a webinar, keep always in mind two lessons; follow the SMART principle and in most cases the simpler the better (Fig. 9.3).

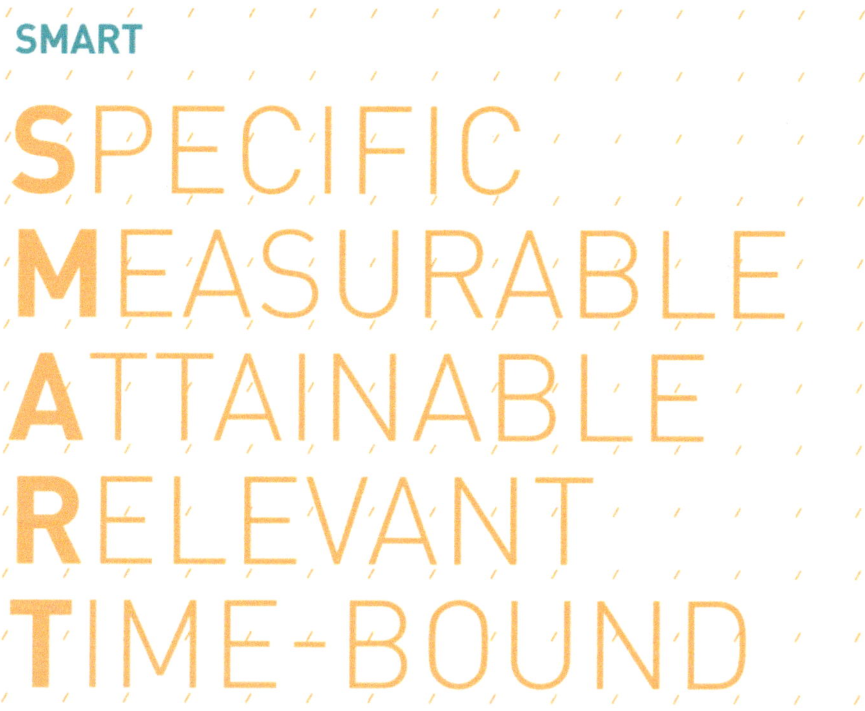

Fig. 9.3 SMART methodology

9.5 The Communication and Promotion

When defining a communication strategy for the webinar, there are key aspects that will lead us to attain our main objective: to make people registered and, more importantly, to have participants. These key aspects can be listed as Who, What, When and How.

1. Who do you want to reach? (Your audience)

   The communication/promotion of a webinar depends on the different target audiences. You will need to tailor the communication strategy to each of those target groups as defined above in "Target Groups" section. Depending on the target audience, you will also need to define the type of channel be used to reach them (i.e. direct emailing, social media, newsletter, press release, etc.).
2. What are you going to tell them? (Your message)

   Ask yourself these questions: "What will motivate or make my target groups participate in my webinar?" "What's in it for them?" "How will they benefit from the information shared in my event?". The way you conceive and communicate your message can help you to achieve your goals and ensure that your message will reach the desired target audiences according to the expected outcome.
3. When are you going to do it? (The timing of your activity)

   Timing is a very important variable. You need to decide very well about the day and hour of your webinar. When deciding the date, you should also always consider if the date chosen for your webinar is a holiday on your target countries, if there are no other major events taking place on that date, to which your target audience may be also interested in, or any other constraints that may affect the registration and participation to your webinar.

   According to the analysis made by GoToWebinar [11] on 250.000 webinars, the best days recommended to organize a webinar are *Wednesday* or *Thursday*. More webinars occur on Wednesdays and Thursdays than any other day of the week, and there is a reason for that, both Wednesday and Thursday have an average attendee count higher than the rest.

   In terms of the time, 10 AM attracts more participants, however, this is a questionable statistic in the case of organizing a webinar with participants from all around the world, because then you will have different hours. Nevertheless, keep this information in mind, 10 AM is the hour where webinars with more participants took place.

   Finally, when you have the date and time decided, start promoting the webinar using the right communication tools/channels.
4. How do you reach your target groups? (The best communication tools/channels to use)

   The tools and channels used will be an essential part of your communication strategy and will influence the outreach of your actions. The use of community-oriented channels is the most efficient way to promote a webinar; this includes social networks and media relations. In order to make the most of social networks, the use of tools like Hootsuite [12], TweetDeck [13], SocialMention [14] and Google Alerts [15] may be considered to facilitate your work and boost the impact of your event.

Have in mind that, when approaching the media through press releases (PR), having strong contacts/relationship with journalists can help in having your content published, otherwise, make sure you search relevant media related to the topic of your webinar and keep the PR clear and to the point.

Another good strategy for communicating your webinar is direct emailing, for this you can use your regular mass mail distribution software or the platforms used for the webinar have features for email distribution, reminders and follow-up. In either case, make sure you comply with the General Data Protection Regulation (GDPR) [16].

Other useful recommendations deriving from the analysis made by GoToWebinar [11] on 250.000 webinars, are the following:

9.5.1 *Start Promoting Early and Steadily*

Promoting the webinar at least 4 weeks in advance results in 12% more registrations on average. But the week leading up to your webinar is when promotion matters most, so make sure you intensify your promotion efforts. Also, don't start promoting it too early, as this may lead to lack of interest.

9.5.2 *Tuesday Is the Best Day to Promote*

When promoting the webinar, this analysis reveals that Tuesdays are the day of the week when more people registers to webinars. Together, Monday, Tuesday and Wednesday attract 63% of all registrations. So, you should avoid sending out invitations or do promotional campaigns on Sundays or Saturdays, and you'll probably may want to skip Friday too.

9.5.3 *Send Emails in the Morning*

While the best time of the day to promote may vary per channel, there is a tendency for registrations between 8 and 10 am. Therefore, sending emails and starting the campaigns early in the morning (always taking into account the time differences from where your participants may come from) may be a good strategy.

9.6 The Content

Webinars should be engaging, short, interesting and to the point, meaning speakers should avoid using overcomplicated explanations about their work. Speakers can use supporting material such as power point presentations, to help the audience to follow the content presented. Depending on the research topic of the webinar the content may vary, but keep in mind using examples or case studies and graph/images to grab the attention. The use of a short video can also be an ice breaker or to rebuild the attention span.

Webinars are also extremely convenient for improving, adjusting, adapting the content, because they can be shared with hundreds of people across the world, including experts, providing a sense of community that is vital for successful, long-lasting communication of the research. Webinars can help researchers, organisations and projects to build a larger audience and database of contacts that can be useful for follow up and future collaborations. Guests can also serve as new contacts that can bring in new audiences, especially if they have their own followers. Webinars can keep audiences engaged long after the live streaming if they are repeatedly posted, shared and promoted online. This enables to have a greater reach because those who couldn't attend the live event are able to watch it afterwards.

Thus, don't forget to record the webinar for future reference and also making it available online to increase the number of viewers.

9.7 The Tools

Webinars are an extremely cost-effective communication, promotional, mentoring and coaching solution. In most cases, all you need is an internet connection and a computer with microphone and camera.

Remember, when people are watching your webinar, they are at their desks in front of a computer so they may be tempted to open other websites, check emails or continue with other work while you are speaking. To keep people engaged, use poll questions, slide decks, and images to enable your audience to interact regularly.

Therefore, the selection of the best software to organise your webinar is of paramount importance and could make the difference between a successful and engaging webinar against something that could be less effective. Although most of the platforms nowadays share the same type of features and functionalities, these can have differences in usability, navigation and appearance. You may have preference of one over the others. Furthermore, the platforms may also have different price-range depending on the functionalities and the number of participants allowed to be hosted that you are looking for, so it is always worth to take a look into a few options and what they have to offer.

Nowadays, there are dozens of tools for organising a webinar, the table below summarises some of them. This list is not exhaustive and intends to be a reference for some of the tools and not influence your decision (Fig. 9.4).

	GoToWebinar	https://www.goto.com/pt/webinar
	BigMarker	https://www.bigmarker.com/
	Zoom	https://zoom.us/
	WebinarNinja	https://webinarninja.com/
	Cisco Webex	https://www.webex.com/
join me	Join.me	https://www.join.me/
	Zoho Meeting	https://www.zoho.com/meeting/
BUSINESS HANGOUTS	Business Hangouts	https://business-hangouts.com/
Microsoft Teams	Microsoft Teams	https://www.microsoft.com/en-us/microsoft-365/microsoft-teams/online-meeting
	Adobe connect	https://www.adobe.com/products/adobeconnect.html

Fig. 9.4 List of webinar tools

9.8 Follow-Up

If you want to make a follow-up action after the webinar, such as downloading a document or take a survey, you need to be clear and make it easy to understand for the participants. Therefore, you should inform the participants about this action/request during the webinar itself and provide the direct links at the webinar and in the follow-up email. Some of the follow-up actions that you can use are as follows.

9.8.1 Ask to Fill in a Feedback Form

As one of the common goals is to gain feedback from our peers and other experts, a brief survey can be sent to the participants ideally on the same day, so that they can provide precious information that can be used as basis for further developments, alterations and improvement.

9.8.2 *Send Additional Content to the Participants*

After the webinar, you can follow up with the participants by sending them additional content via email. People who registered but did not show up or left the webinar earlier can be included and receive this content as well, as this action can also encourage them to (fully) participate the next time.

9.8.3 *Send Follow-Up Email to Absentees*

You may consider to send a follow-up email to the registered people that didn't show up at the webinar. In that email you may send some conclusions and also a link to the recorded session, if you have it (this is something we strongly advice). As mentioned above, this may encourage them to participate in other future webinars.

9.9 Final Remarks and Conclusions

It is through times like these that we truly show our ability to change and adapt. One of the greatest examples of overcoming the constrains caused by the COVID-19 is *Le Tour de France virtuel*. In the context of the health crisis in which the majority of cycling events were cancelled the organisers have set up a virtual riding using ZWIFT [17] that was watched live on TV by thousands of viewers. Even that this is not an official tour, it shows how the current status of technology, our ability to adapt to the circumstances and our drive to have a new normal.

The same happens in science communication, these days without any precedents in the modern era, we need to reinvent the way we communicate. Webinars are a great example of how we can deliver high impactful events. I dare even to say that the webinars are here to stay stronger than ever, prevailing as a simpler and more cost-effective way to present scientific achievements and knowledge.

Acknowledgements We would like to acknowledge the participation of the LOBA teams in the support to the creation of this chapter, especially the European Project department personified in the people of Candela Bravo, Catarina Pereira, Pietro Rigonat and Raquel Nogueira.

References

1. Guide to science and medical communication. https://www.mastersincommunications.com/.
2. https://www.webex.com.
3. https://www.gotomeeting.com/.
4. https://clickmeeting.com/.

5. https://myownconference.com/.
6. Learn how to reach your target groups. 2017 Dandelion Project. http://www.dandelion-europe.eu.
7. https://www.mentimeter.com/.
8. https://www.lift-bbi.eu/webinars/events/webinar-4-value-chains-and-innovation-ecosystem/.
9. https://www.lift-bbi.eu/.
10. Science communication: a visual perspective. 2019; Yael Fitzpatrick. https://www.aldacenter.org/aklc/webinars/visual-perspective.
11. Big book of webinar stats: we analyzed 250,000 webinars to help you make yours better.
12. https://hootsuite.com/.
13. https://tweetdeck.twitter.com/.
14. http://socialmention.com/.
15. https://www.google.com/alerts.
16. https://gdpr.eu/compliance/.
17. https://www.zwift.com/.

Chapter 10
The Virtual Theater: The Lure, the Title, the Scene, the Backstage, and the Space

Andrew Juurinen

10.1 Introduction

10.1.1 The Demands to Connect with Colleagues Are Evolving

Succeeding in the medical sciences is not for the faint of heart—it requires a tremendous amount of dedication and hard work and its only getting harder. Staying on top of current research is a challenge; statistics indicate that the number of scientific papers that are published increases yearly by 8–9% [1], which makes it difficult to keep up to date with reading requirements.

Moreover, it is generally accepted that competition for funding and placements in the medical sciences has increased over several decades. Today's medical scientists must navigate through a competitive landscape of grant proposals, conferences, reviews, lectures, networking events, in addition to reading or writing research papers. Trying to complete these requirements in isolation may not be the answer. Instead, connecting with colleagues and peers to expand personal networks and to discover or share content as a group may be essential to success in the field. By using journal clubs, curated social media feeds, blogs, webinars, conferences, and additional touchpoints, some scientists are finding ways to connect with colleagues to better cope with the demands of this field [1].

As lockdown measures imposed by governments continue globally in response to the COVID-19 pandemic, a growing number of scientific conferences are being cancelled [2]. As a result, one of the best-known ways to expand networks and to promote scientific work is being rapidly extinguished. Over and above the pressure to cancel these in-person events, many scientists are becoming cognizant of the

A. Juurinen (✉)
Xtalks, Part of Honeycomb Worldwide Inc., Toronto, Canada
e-mail: ajuurinen@xtalks.com

G. C. Di Renzo (ed.), *Essential Writing, Communication and Narrative Skills for Medical Scientists Before and After the COVID Era*,
https://doi.org/10.1007/978-3-030-84954-2_10

enormous carbon footprint that physical conferences and tradeshows are responsible for and are beginning to evaluate the need for such events [3–6].

In response, webinar events have filled this gap and are being used as an exceptional tool to promote scientific work, debate peers, exchange new ideas and market new products or services [7]. As more scientists begin to fully realize webinar technology as a meaningful scientific communication tool, competition here too will reign. Within the scope of this competitive landscape, scientists who adopt the mindset of a brand may be the best positioned to succeed.

10.1.2 Considering the Scientist as a Brand

Succeeding in the medical science field means scientists must not only keep up with the scientific work of peers but also find ways of promoting their own work. As these new ways of sharing information have blossomed over the last decade, researchers may have learned that the subject of marketing is no longer a domain that should solely be studied by those in the business field.

From a self-promotion perspective, to gain a greater reach and to further a career in the medical sciences, scientists (whether they are aware of this or not) have needed to develop a marketing skill set. Whether the ultimate goal of the scientist is to win a grant proposal, to acquire a new job, or to sell their amazing new technology, knowing the fundamentals of marketing is key to getting their work found, read, understood, sold, and cited [8]. If scientists are viewing their own work as a brand that should be consumed, then adopting a marketing skill set is essential.

10.1.3 Webinars as a Meaningful Touchpoint

The concept of a consumer touchpoint is one of the most basic concepts that is introduced when learning the fundamentals of marketing. Touchpoints are the interactions where a consumer, or in the case of a medical scientist, a peer group, makes contact with a scientist's work. If more touchpoints are available to the peer group, there is a greater chance that a scientist's work can be discovered.

In addition to the touchpoints mentioned above (Sect. 10.1.1), the number and types of platforms available for consuming scientific information have increased dramatically over the last decade. From search engines like Google Scholar and Mendeley, which help researchers discover and curate the latest research, to platforms like Genbank and Github, which help scientists organize and share data, the number of ways to connect with fellow scientists seems endless [9–12].

With that said, webinars offer a platform to openly discuss, integrate, and share many of the touchpoints listed above, within a model that allows for easily accessible, real-time, and peer-to-peer discussion. Much like speaking at a scientific conference, webinars offer opportunities to create excitement around scientific efforts by creating an event which is solely dedicated to a specific topic. In ways that written work cannot convey, webinars are offering scientists a forum to reveal unpublished data, create greater context, as well as convey a passion, authenticity, and personality to their work.

As you will discover in this chapter, webinars offer features that can accelerate a new way forward for scientific communications. This chapter begins with "The Lure" (Sect. 10.2) which further discusses why webinars are a worthy scientific communication tool and will outline general methods used to drive attendance. A discussion of the "The Title" (Sect. 10.3) and "The Scene" (Sect. 10.4) will describe best practices for constructing webinar content with respect to webinar titles and event pages. "The Backstage" (Sect. 10.5) will discuss the features of webinar platforms that offer organizers ways of optimizing their interactions with audience members prior to and during a live webinar. "The Space" (Sect. 10.6) will offer insights on optimizing presentation value for the audience and will outline several presentation formats that best work in a webinar context. A prediction about the future of webinars as a communication tool will conclude the discussion (Sect. 10.7). After reading this chapter, you will develop a strong understanding of how webinars may best function as a tool to augment the reach of your scientific efforts.

10.2 The Lure

10.2.1 Using Webinars as a Means to Entice an Audience

Market research forecasts that the global webinar market will expand at a compound annual growth rate of 7.6% between 2016 and 2023 [13]. This is due to many factors, including that technology in this field seems to be improving year-over-year as more audiences are exposed to learning via a webinar platform. In this section, an outline will be given of why webinars are inherently an important tool to disseminate scientific information and how they can entice an audience to engage with content.

10.2.2 A Live Event Worthy of Interest

Webinars are an effective tool to encourage excitement around a scientific topic simply because they offer a structured event that is held at a specific time and place. The inherent nature of an event offers something that is newsworthy to the online consumer [14]. Although many webinars offer recorded versions of their live event, once the webinar has ended, the opportunity to be part of the live event has passed, and more importantly, webinar presenters are no longer available to interact with the attendees in real time. Thus, if webinar registrants are interested in these aspects of participation, they are more likely to attend the live event. In addition, because of the ease with which webinars are shared through scientific peer groups, individuals may feel an increased obligation or desire to attend in an effort to further connect with their immediate scientific community.

10.2.3 Timeliness

One of the greatest advantages to webinars over in-person events is their ability to be held and promoted on short notice. If a new scientific development occurs or important data is released, scientists may quickly connect with their audience to communicate their thoughts or clarify the impacts of this new data. Webinars may be shared or even live-streamed on social platforms during the event itself, thereby giving immediate live access to potentially interested colleagues on extremely short notice [15].

10.2.4 Accessibility

Since webinars do not require the travel time that is necessary to attend a physical conference, the potential audience who is interested in the topic will be more likely to attend the event. Instead of dedicating several days to a specific event or speaking engagement, webinar participants only require a relatively small amount time for attendance. From a productivity perspective, this makes webinars vastly superior to in-person events. Recordings of webinars are often made available for registrants unable to attend the live event. Additionally, costs that are typically associated with in-person events such as a transportation, lodging, and food are no longer required, when attending a webinar.

Since only an internet connection and a computer (or mobile device) are needed for access, webinars have opened up the barriers that are typically associated with talks held at physical conferences. Thus, the audience and speakers may be connecting to the webinar from multiple geographical locations around the world. This also implies that webinar participants may join from several continents and time zones simultaneously.

10.2.5 Interactivity

Similar to in-person events, many webinars offer a question and answer session during the presentation. The opportunity to ask questions and receive real-time answers is something that provides value. Having real-time access to peers and their scientific work is in many ways much better than reading a colleague's article or downloading their shared data set. This access to the speaker's insights about the details of their presentation can be invaluable to both the webinar attendee and to the presenters themselves.

A question and answer session offers additional opportunities to help the speaker clarify their research and communicate it in a way that is most valuable to the webinar audience. Webinars also offer additional ways to interact with the audience, such as live audience polling and pre- or post-webinar surveys. These additional touchpoints can be advantageous for both the webinar presenters and the audience members. For presenters, receiving audience feedback prior to the event via webinar registration forms helps to identify questions about their research and sometimes offers perspectives on where to guide the focus of their presentation.

During the event, polling questions offer real-time feedback or opinions that can help to facilitate discussions or highlight points of interest. Post-webinar surveys also provide presenters with feedback on their presentation and can help guide them on topics for future presentations. For webinar attendees, these types of interactions offer an enhanced experience, allowing a greater perceived accessibility to the speaker, and are typically unavailable during in-person speaking engagements.

10.2.6 Reduced Carbon Footprint

Increases in global carbon emissions are expected to cause devastating and lasting negative impacts on economic well-being, health, and food security [16–18]. Research has shown that a three-day, 1000-person national conference can generate more than 580 tons of CO_2 emissions every year, and for certain conferences, the amount of CO_2 emissions can be several fold greater [19]. An estimate of the 2014 Society for Neuroscience Conference, for example, indicates that over 22,000 metric tons of CO_2 were produced as a result of the physical event [4]. As the negative impact of physical conferences' carbon footprints continue to be highlighted within the scientific community, organizers are turning to online meetings as a more efficient, viable, and carbon-friendly alternative [6].

10.2.7 Driving Webinar Attendance

Although content choices (e.g., webinar title and webinar abstracts) are extremely important when attempting to increase webinar attendance, this next section will discuss which additional marketing techniques can best drive webinar registrations.

10.2.7.1 Using Existing Webinar Service Providers

When planning to host a webinar, there are two general options to choose from. Individuals or organizations either can personally host, market, and produce their own webinar or can choose an existing service provider to help market and produce their webinar. If one chooses to personally host the webinar using an existing software platform, the organizer must rely on their existing network and marketing resources to encourage registrations [20, 21]. When choosing this first option, it will be important to make use of the digital marketing techniques outlined in the next section.

In the medical science community, there are a wide range of service providers available, including academic groups, societies and associations, and commercial service providers [22–24]. Choosing an existing webinar service provider generally eases the responsibility of marketing the webinar to an interested audience. Depending on the goals of the individuals or organization looking to hold this webinar, access to the above service providers may be limited due to policy or funding. In general, commercial organizations that wish to speak, present, or sponsor a webinar typically require financial payment to the webinar service provider [25].

Choosing an existing webinar service provider allows presenters to expand their existing network by using the marketing services of this provider, but does not necessarily limit the ability of the webinar presenters to leverage their own networks and marketing outlets.

Employing Digital Marketing Strategies

In general, generic lead-generation marketing strategies can be applied to webinar event pages, assuming that the goal of the presenters is to reach a maximum number of webinar registrants. For the purposes of this chapter, a high-level overview of several traffic channels will be discussed.

Email

One of the most obvious but effective methods to generate interest in a webinar is to send an email about the webinar to a list of potential registrants. The subject line and preheader text of the email should aim to engage the potential participant with a clear message as to the content of the webinar itself. To be effective, the email content should detail obvious elements like the date and time of the webinar [26].

Perhaps less obvious, for those who typically attend or organize physical conferences, is a listing of alternative date and time zone information for potential webinar participants who wish to connect from other time zones throughout the globe [27]. Email content typically includes the title of the event, a shortened version of what will be discussed during the webinar, and a listing of the webinar presenter(s). Finally, a link to the webinar event page should be included.

Including too little or too much information can be problematic for generating traffic to the webinar event page [26]. In addition to simply inviting individuals to a webinar, email is also the primary method used to remind successful registrants to attend the live webinar (SMS-based reminders and phone call-based reminders are also used) [28]. Webinar reminder emails are often a built-in feature of many webinar platforms and are generally accepted to increase the live attendance rate [26].

Organic Traffic

By strategically focusing on keywords or key phrases in the construction of a webinar event page, one is able to increase the visibility of this page in search engine results. By doing so, it is possible to convert a proportion of that traffic into webinar registrations. This search engine optimization (SEO) technique is typically part of a larger domain-wide strategy but can also be applied to individual webpages. Although the details of these strategies are debated among so-called SEO experts, incorporating the keyword or keyphrase in the URL, H1 tag, meta-description, and alt image tags on a webpage are common techniques to improve search engine visibility [29] .

Referral Traffic

To truly optimize the organic traffic channel, hyperlinks from domains outside of the webinar event page must connect to the webpage. These types of hyperlinks are known as referral links or backlinks. As the number of backlinks accumulate, depending on a number of factors, including search query and link quality, search engines may begin to populate the webinar event page closer to the top of the search results. Thus, backlinks aid in attaining a higher search position in search returns and, of course, driving web-traffic from the hyperlinked page itself [30].

Webinar backlinks can be built by a coordinated outreach campaign, either by asking those involved to hyperlink to the webinar using their own domains or asking outside of one's personal network. Generally, if the quality of content in the webinar is of interest to an audience, backlinks will organically accumulate.

Social Media

With the omnipresence of social media on the web, it is prudent to utilize social media channels to promote the webinar. To maximize reach on social media, a coordinated approach from webinar presenters and organizers is optimal. With this type of approach, a particular social media post can be given the maximum possible number of interactions, thereby giving it the opportunity for greater visibility across personal social networks [31]. Several social media posts or messages about the webinar, across a timeframe prior to the webinar, will also help to maximize visibility. There are a wide number of social media platforms now available. In North America, it may be worthwhile to focus efforts on those that are typically considered "popular," like LinkedIn and Twitter, within the medical scientific community [32].

That said, if time dedicated to posting across social media channels is a consideration, there are several programs available to consolidate your social media posting efforts and minimize the amount of time necessary to post across a wider variety of channels [33, 34]. When doing so, using relevant hashtags used by the community and posting in related community channels is recommended [35]. As with referral hyperlinks, if the quality of the webinar content and title is appealing to an audience, organic shares of the webinar event page may begin to accumulate on individual social media accounts. These may occur either through sharing of the webinar event page directly or through the resharing of social posts that were previously written.

Webinar Referrals

Visitors to a webinar event page can be prompted at some point in the registration process to refer a colleague to the webinar. This can be done at any point during the interaction with the webinar registration's content, including on the webinar registration page itself (sometimes assisted through a web automation) or when registrants first receive their confirmation of registration email [36].

Since those who register for the webinar are likely the most interested and engaged individuals (i.e., the correct target audience), their immediate network of colleagues may also be interested in attending. These referrals can also occur during a webinar itself [37]. Similar to referral hyperlinks and social media shares, direct shares of the webinar are more likely to occur when the webinar registrants are intrigued by its high-quality content. Although not considered a digital marketing strategy, referrals can also occur by word-of-mouth among colleagues and are worth acknowledging as a viable, but unreliable, method of driving webinar registrations.

Paid

If there is a budget available to promote a webinar, developing a paid marketing campaign can be a very effective way to increase webinar registrations [38]. Paid campaigns can be organized through a wide range of advertising platforms. To display webinar advertisements, search engine advertising platforms may be used to target specific areas of interest in search returns [39]. Display network platforms offer advertisements for display on partner websites as banners [40]. Social media platforms offer advertising options within the social platforms themselves and sometimes within partner networks as display advertisements [38]. Because medical science webinars are typically highly specific with regard to their content and target audience, it is best to use advertising platforms that are capable of targeting a unique audience. This can mean, restricting audiences by their associated keywords, job titles, organizations, and interests.

10.3 The Title

Before a webinar title is even considered, a webinar topic must first be decided upon. A non-scientific or casual review of webinar topics in the medical sciences reveals a wide-ranging series of topics, and it is beyond the scope of this chapter to offer any guidance about which scientific topics are best suited for webinars. However, from experience, there are several generalities that can be formed to give guidance on the types of topics that appear to be the most popular with registrants. That said, a thorough review of topics and registration rates are needed to confirm this guidance. In general, these topics include:

1. New method, service, or product developments that may impact the medical sciences.
2. Regulatory developments that impact the medical sciences industry.
3. Reviews or analyses of medical science topics.
4. Presentations of recent journal article publications.
5. Discussions of other news-worthy events.

Creating an intriguing topic for a webinar can first begin with an understanding of your target audience. What are their job titles? What types of problems are they experiencing? If webinar organizers are able to gain the perspective of their potential audience, this may help to influence the decision-making process. Evaluating whether or not your audience would want to attend the topic of choice is a better approach than covering a topic simply because it serves your interests.

Once a general topic is chosen, selecting a title is often the next step. This is understood to be one of the most important factors to consider when trying to acquire registrants for a webinar [41]. Webinar titles are front-and-center in most shared hyperlinks, due to coded meta-tags that allow previews of webpage titles, descriptions, and images on most platforms [42]. Webinar titles are also displayed in webinar invitations, social posts, website listings, invitations, paid campaigns, search engine results, and of course on the webinar event page itself. Optimally, the title should aim to describe the purpose of the webinar and why a potential registrant might want to attend and to avoid any jargon-laden language [43].

As mentioned in the previous section, incorporating keywords in the title is essential to SEO efforts. These specific keywords, when placed in the title, help to drive web traffic from search engines and can assist in improving search engine results [29].

In terms of title length, it is recommended to keep titles under 70 characters long [44]. An analysis of life science webinar conversion rates revealed that there was no correlation between the number of registrations and webinar title character lengths. Keeping titles under 70 characters long ensures that when these titles appear in search engine results, the full title is displayed and not truncated [45]. Keeping titles untruncated has been shown to increase the number of clicks on webpages [44]. Moreover, any shares of the webinar event page that may populate its title using meta tags may also truncate the webinar title if titles are not kept under 70 characters [46]. Thus, keeping titles of this length may ultimately get more views of your webinar event page.

10.4 The Scene

When a title and topic is engaging enough, potential registrants may then read the webinar abstract to get more details about the webinar itself to decide if they should register. Typically, a webinar event page contains the content of the webinar, the speakers involved, and either the webinar registration form itself or a hyperlink to a separate the registration form. Ultimately, this is the last item of content that should aim to convert viewers of this page into webinar registrants.

Webinars are intended to be a scheduled time commitment of typically between 30 and 90 minutes. Online conferences which often contain multiple webinar sessions require even more of a time commitment, as sometimes they may be held over a period of several days. Unlike a journal article abstract, webinar abstracts must convey to potential webinar registrants why they should dedicate a significant portion of their day to attend the live webinar. To contrast with journal article abstracts, which will often summarize the details of the methods used, results, and conclusions of the research, webinar abstracts are best constructed to simply hint at these points.

10.4.1 Tips for Writing a Webinar Abstract

When committing to write the content of the webinar abstract, it may be beneficial to break the abstract into five components. This approach aims to optimize the conversion of your webinar event page viewers into actual webinar registrants. The tips in this section for writing abstracts have been primarily surmised from a review of thousands of abstracts and their resulting webinar attendance.

Firstly, maintaining a voice that focuses on the reader or the problems that a reader might be experiencing may be helpful in this conversion. This can begin with a statement of the problem upon which your research was focused. What latent issue or problem was trying to be fixed or addressed by the research or scientific work?

How does that apply to the reader? Recognizing the issues or pain-points of your reader are a key to the opening component of a webinar abstract [47].

The second component of an optimal abstract addresses how the issues raised in the first component will be explained during the webinar. This section of the abstract can be a short explanation of what will be addressed in the webinar. These two opening components alone could serve as a complete understanding of why readers should register for a webinar.

A third component will build upon what was stated in the first two components by outlining interesting and supportive facts about the presented content, helping to solidify the topics that will be addressed during the webinar to ultimately build interest for the reader in said topic [47].

The fourth component is a direct explanation of what readers will learn if they attend the webinar. This can be constructed in either sentences or a bulleted list.

Finally, a call-to-action serves as a final reminder to readers that they need to take action and register for the event. If additional webinar assets are included in the live presentation, such as whitepapers, articles, or data sets, the call-to-action can showcase this final offer as a reason to register for the webinar.

Research shows that an abstract's length can be an important factor in converting readers into webinar registrants [45]. Measuring the number of words or characters in a webinar abstract revealed that shorter abstracts yield higher reader-to-webinar registrant conversion rates. With that said, one should take into consideration SEO opportunities so that the webinar event page may appear in a search engine result. Research also reveals that if word count is too low on the webpage, it may not optimally appear in a search engine result page [48].

That said, measuring the content length of webpages is a contested SEO variable [49, 50], so it may be prudent to assume that extremely small abstracts may not perform as well in search engine results as longer form abstracts. If the aims of a webinar event page are to drive as much relevant traffic to a webpage as possible and to convert as much of that traffic into webinar registrants as possible, then a balanced approach to abstract length is recommended. This means a balance between smaller abstract length, to optimize viewer-to-webinar conversions, and a minimum content length to ensure potential search visibility. Functionally, 300 words in length is a recommendation, but more research would be needed to validate the data across multiple domains [45].

10.4.2 Additional Components of a Webinar Event Page

Including the date and time of the webinar across multiple time zones can help to clarify webinar start times in different geographical locations and can act to limit scheduling conflicts. As alluded to earlier in this chapter, a notice declaring that a recording of the webinar is available to registrants may help to increase overall webinar registrations.

Considering that colored visuals may increase an individual's willingness to read a piece of content significantly [51], the use of images and other graphic design constructs on the webinar event page may also help to increase the conversion of webpage visitors to webinar registrants. Since opinions about webpages can be formed rapidly, research indicates that the use of imagery, design choices, and webpage structure may facilitate a good impression about the webpage in general—in about 50 milliseconds [52–54].

The use of multiple speakers is generally accepted to be a best practice when conducting a webinar [55]. Including more than one speaker in a webinar gives the opportunity for multiple speakers to share and invite their own network of peers to the event [56]. In addition, inviting several speakers from a diverse set of organizations may offer the impression that the webinar's content is more dynamic and could deliver greater insights than those of a sole speaker. Taken together, these points indicate that inviting more than one speaker may benefit the webinar as a whole. Webinar event pages often include speaker's names, titles, and a short biography [57, 58].

10.5 The Backstage

Choosing the best webinar platform for your application can be a daunting process. The number of webinar platforms available may seem overwhelming, and a thorough review of all available platforms may not be feasible. Each webinar platform may have slightly different features but will have a core functionality that will remain the same. Most of these components are configurable behind the scenes and will be discussed in the remainder of this chapter.

10.5.1 Registration

Webinar platforms will provide a means of registering individuals for the webinar, using field choices like email and name, as well as optional choices like job title, organization, and phone number. It is generally accepted by marketers that reducing the number of fields will increase the number of webpage form conversions [59]. As such, it is important for webinar organizers to decide which information is critical to capture during the webinar registration process and which information can be left out to maximize the conversion rate. Since receiving pre-event feedback or demographics can help to solidify the focus of a presentation, webinar organizers should determine what is most important before implementing additional required fields.

Once users sign up for a webinar, successful registrants can be sent a confirmation of registration via email, as well as reminders about the webinar [60]. These emails will function to give registrants a hyperlink to access the live webinar and other information like audio options, date, and time reminders.

A note about privacy:
If the intentions of the webinar organizer(s) are to further communicate marketing content or share webinar registrant information with third parties, webinar registration forms may need to include disclaimer or opt-in agreement clauses. These can include either a statement indicating that registrants agree to the disclaimer terms by registering for the webinar or may give attendees an option to be included in (or excluded from) additional marketing communications.
These legal requirements are in place to protect users' data privacy and are becoming a growing concern for marketers in general. With the introduction of the General Data Protection Regulation in May of 2018 in Europe, and with the more recent enactment of the California Consumer Privacy Act in January 2020 [61], webinar organizers need to understand how these legislations affect the way in which they collect, store, and document personal data of webinar registrants.
While the complexities of these legislations are beyond the scope of this chapter, it is important to note that when organizers obtain personal information from data subjects who are protected under these legislations, they must comply with these laws or face severe financial penalties [62].

10.5.2 The Green Room

Most webinar platforms offer a feature where organizers and speakers can communicate with each other, without being audible to the audience, prior to the live broadcast. This "green room" can be used to decide exactly who is presenting and when, how presentation slides will be displayed, how a question and answer session might be facilitated, and more [63].

Time spent in the green room should be used to determine if speaker's audio quality is satisfactory and if webcams are being used, how to optimize these video feeds. Since time is often limited before the agreed upon start time of the broadcast, webinar presenters need to plan enough in advance to account for this preparation period.

10.5.3 Sharing Content During the Webinar

Depending on the webinar platform, webinar presentations may be shared through a number of different methods. When considering that most presentations will use presentation slides in some form, a presentation slide deck may be uploaded to the webinar platform so that several presenters may share the same presentation slide deck at the same time. This requires that presentations are typically uniform in dimensions and finished prior to the broadcast for upload [64].

Other types of webinar platforms offer a screen sharing function so that webinar presenters can share anything that they can display on their computer screens, including Microsoft Powerpoint presentations, Microsoft Excel sheets, websites, and more. Screen sharing platforms also allow in-session edits to presentation files and differences in webinar slide dimensions.

10.5.4 Webcams

Most modern webinar platforms also offer the ability for presenters to display a webcam for their presentation. Best practices indicate that speakers should keep their camera at eye-level, keep eye contact with the camera when speaking, avoid backlighting, use soft-front lighting, and be conscious of their background setting [65]. These settings should be optimized in the webinar green room (Sect. 10.5.2). There may be a benefit to using a webcam since it has been demonstrated that speech recognition is improved when a listener can visualize a human face when compared to audio alone [66].

When considering a multiple-speaker scenario in the absence of a webcam, evidence suggests that there will be longer pauses between speaker interactions due to the absence of paralinguistic cues, which help identify when to speak. This would indicate that in an effort to keep the conversation fluid, it may be best to use webcams. That said, evidence also suggests that the perceived benefits of a video feed in a pedagogical scenario may not necessary lead to improved learning [67].

10.5.5 Additional Webinar Assets

Many webinar platforms also offer methods of distributing hyperlinks or handouts which can contain a wide variety of different file types. Hyperlinks can direct audience members to other supporting presentation assets or prompts to register for organizer initiatives. Files may include items like the webinar slide deck, additional data sets, whitepapers, and journal articles.

Video files are also sometimes included as a handout for viewing as a download after the webinar [68]. However, videos may also be displayed during the webinar itself for all viewers and audience members to watch concurrently.

In contrast, at a physical conference, these types of assets are typically not as easily available to audience members. Instead, papers or pamphlets can be used, but may ultimately be discarded. By having these webinar assets immediately available on audience members' personal devices, this can result in more views or interactions with any handouts, hyperlinks or videos added to the webinar.

10.5.6 Using Poll Questions

Webinar poll questions are real-time, live opinion surveys of the audience. Incorporating the use of poll questions during a webinar is a way of getting the audience to interact with a presenter's content and can also serve as a short 1–2 min break from the main presentation.

Webinar polling questions can be used in multiple ways to facilitate discussion and interaction during a webinar. Research indicates that some form of active learning, while integrated with passive learning can have benefits in a classroom setting [69]. Webinar poll questions offer an active learning opportunity for the webinar audience. Poll results can be displayed on a live broadcast so audience members can learn the opinions of their peers, while comparing against their own poll answers.

Hosts can incorporate the answers of a live poll in their presentation to shift the focus of their presentation to something that is most relatable to the live audience. For example, if a webinar presenter learned that the majority of their audience had experience in a particular subject matter, they could steer their presentation to focus on that topic.

Polling questions can also be used as a testing tool to act as a teaching aid. Test results can be obtained from individual poll answers and may be reported back to host to evaluate the audience's knowledge.

Future webinar content ideas can also be derived from polling questions. Asking the audience directly about what they would like to learn in a future webinar is a way of building a relationship with the audience and may help to maintain a consistent and growing audience throughout a webinar series.

10.5.7 Audience Questions and Internal Chats

Most webinar platforms include a chat function within the webinar software interface so that audience members or organizers can submit questions or comments among themselves without disrupting the audio feed of the webinar. Questions relating to webinar technical problems or questions that can be answered by non-presenters can be addressed more quickly with additional webinar administrative support staff using this chat feature. In addition, because this allows for the submission of questions throughout a presentation, audience members do not need to wait and hold their questions until the question and answer session arrives.

Certain webinar platforms also allow free chat discussions among audience members during the presentation and can help facilitate an environment that encourages audience collaboration without disrupting the primary presentation.

Alternatively, unlike during an in-person question and answer period, webinar question and answer sessions may be moderated in a private channel. This channel can be shared among speakers, organizers and webinar assistants who can screen the best questions that are submitted from the audience [70]. Webinar organizers have found benefit from using private chats to either eliminate non-relevant questions from the audience or help to facilitate a panel-style scenario, by privately discussing how to get less vocal panelists to answer on certain audience questions [6].

Most webinar platforms also offer some form of webinar data reporting that may include all written conversations or questions that were submitted during the webinar [71]. For some presentations, more questions may be asked than can be answered during the live broadcast time, so webinar reports are a way for organizers to follow up with all submissions. Depending on the contact information supplied by the audience member, organizers may follow up with these questions or discussions via email or phone call.

10.5.8 Post-Webinar Survey

Similar to the webinar registration form, post-webinar surveys are available to organizers and can be used to acquire feedback from the audience [72]. These can be launched for audience members when the webinar closes. The questions created in the post-webinar survey can help hosts understand how to better improve future webinars by asking the audience to rate or comment on the content that was presented.

10.5.9 Webinar Data Reporting

Any webinar information collected during the webinar registration process and live broadcast may be included in a post-webinar data report. Group results such as attendance percentage or average time spent in a webinar can be derived from combining data from all participants. Individual audience member data is also commonly reported during a webinar. This can include data such as polling answer submissions, question submissions, number of handouts downloaded, and time entered and exited data [71]. Webinar interest scores are also common among various platforms. Webinar interest scores can be calculated by assigning a value to the time spent within the webinar application and interactions with poll questions or chat features in the interface [73].

In general, webinar data reports offer many ways for webinar organizers to learn how the webinar registrants engaged with the content and help to serve as a benchmark for future webinars. For commercial organizations, webinar data reports give access to registrant contact information and can serve as a means for lead generation.

10.6 The Space

10.6.1 Connecting to the Audience with Structure

When beginning to construct the webinar presentation itself, it may be useful to ask several questions. What is the goal of the presentation? For medical scientists, the goals are typically either to communicate the results of scientific work or to build relationships with prospective or existing clients and investors. Whether the goal is to outline research findings or present a commercial offering, advice for presentation content is similar—simplify the story, incorporate some amount of detail and data, while maintaining a thread of the key takeaways and story narrative throughout [74].

Marketing initiatives that target scientists should highlight a product or service's unique value that differentiates it in the marketplace. David Chapman who authored a book on marketing in the life sciences offers this advice—identify the uniqueness of an offering, articulate the differences, test the claims made, and promote those claims through various marketing touchpoints [75]. Focusing on the needs of the audience rather than a detailed description of the product or service should also be an aim for any webinars with a commercial intent [76].

When deciding on the structure of the presentation, it has been said that the most compelling presentations use a structure that alternatingly juxtaposes *what is* (the current state of affairs) and *what could be* (the potential for the future). Employing this type of conflict and resolution narrative throughout a presentation has been documented in what are perceived as the most powerful presentations [77]. Typically, these presentations include a defined beginning, middle and end, with a call-to-action. For webinars, this call-to-action could mean any initiative that could elicit meaningful interaction. This could be a commercial service inquiry, a download of a journal article, or an invitation to collaborate.

10.6.2 Considerations for Audio and Visual

When deciding how to orally communicate the webinar, presenters may choose to memorize or read from a prewritten script, or memorize the key points when delivering the details of the presentation. Generally, most speakers are not capable of reading from a script and sounding authentic and may lack the ability to connect with the audience in this way [74]. That said, some of the best presentations delivered were scripted, albeit delivered with conviction [78]. Whether to deliver a scripted or unscripted webinar may be a decision best left to presenters based on their comfort level.

When designing slides, presenters should consider outlining just one idea per slide. Slide pacing recommendations are variable, with some experts suggesting a relatively slow pacing of 1–2 min per slide, a moderate pacing of 30–60 s per slide, or even a rapid-fire approach near 20 s per slide (or transition) [77, 79]. Incorporating the use of large fonts with uncluttered text and employing the use of imagery also helps to facilitate a more powerful presentation [54, 77]. The use of presentation slides is, of course, optional, as webcam feeds can be integrated within any type of webinar formats discussed below.

10.6.3 Webinar Formats

Up until this point in the chapter, most of the content has been assuming a single or multi-speaker keynote presentation. Typically, these presentations begin with an introduction by a webinar moderator and an introduction to the speaker. The main component of the presentation follows this and is perhaps interrupted for one or multiple polling questions. To finish this style of presentation, the webinar is concluded with a question and answer session.

Question and answer sessions, as discussed earlier in the chapter, can be moderated by additional staff. Audience questions may be read aloud to the speaker(s), rather than incorporating live audio feeds from the audience. Seed or planted questions that appear as though they have been generated by the audience can help to facilitate discussion at the beginning or throughout the question and answer session if needed.

Engaging with the audience can be difficult for mature presenters who are accustomed to feedback from audience laughter at an in-person presentation. In a webinar, allowing audience audio feeds to be open would likely result in overwhelming audience noise during a live broadcast. While live audio audience feeds may be possible in small virtual groups, there doesn't seem to be a suitable correlate for this type of engagement in a webinar setting.

For presenters hoping for more interaction with the audience, keynote-style presentations should aim to integrate audience questions or comments mid-presentation and make use of polling questions throughout to drive the direction of discussion.

Panel-based webinars or the less formal fireside chat format of webinars are an alternative to the single or multi-speaker keynote style webinar. In this presentation style, a moderator will help to drive conversation through a series of questions asked to multiple speakers. Panel discussions give audience members access to multiple perspectives of what is often a complex and multifaceted topic [80]. In this style, a webinar moderator will need to be well researched and be skilled enough to lead the conversation in a logical and pleasing manner. Audience questions may be integrated throughout or left near the end of the webinar.

Question and answer style webinars can make use of questions submitted by the audience during the webinar registration process. In this format of webinar, the audience is looking to have their own questions drive the conversation, rather than the content of the presentation being decided by the presenters themselves.

Moderators who drive this type of webinar will need to encourage audience members throughout the presentation to submit their questions.

Roundtable format webinars may be used in situations where a traditional webinar audience is not even present and can sometimes be considered a closed virtual meeting. That said, audience members may also be invited to this format of webinar. This type of webinar format may be best to facilitate a forum for problem solving, collaboration, ideas, and sharing of experiences. The aim of this type of format is to have speakers have equal opportunity to share perspectives on a topic. Smaller roundtable sessions can follow traditional webinar panel discussions or keynote presentations in an aim to generate excitement and information exchange based on the primary webinar topic presented.

10.7 Webinar Use as a Scientific Communication Tool in the Future

Whether the goal of hosting a webinar is to promote a research effort or to market a new product launch, webinars are clearly a highly effective means to facilitate communications. More recently, as a result of the COVID-19 pandemic and government-issued lockdown orders, the trend of using webinars continues to emerge [7]. As the number of cancelled tradeshows and conferences increase, medical science marketers will need to fill these gaps in their lead generation efforts, and the use of webinars will allow scientists to continue to communicate their research effectively [6, 7].

With a rise in the number of users participating in these webinars, one would expect that the comfort level and familiarity with webinar technology, as defined in this chapter, should also increase.

As such, the methods used to market webinars and the webinar technology itself will likely evolve in the future. Ultimately, this may lead to even greater use of webinars as a means by which scientific information can be communicated.

Throughout this chapter, webinars were pointed out as a more advantageous communication tool than in-person conferences and tradeshows. In light of physical distancing and lockdown orders during the COVID-19 pandemic, it is possible that the medical science community will embrace webinars as the new normal.

As lockdown measures begin to ease globally, from a carbon-footprint perspective, there is an ever-present reality that remains. Physical conferences and tradeshows are unsustainable [4, 19]. This realization coupled with the impact of the COVID-19 pandemic may serve as a necessary turning point, thereby paving a path for webinars to emerge as a primary communication platform for medical scientists.

This transition from in-person events to webinars may be rebutted by several factors. Conference companies may resume the production of their existing in-person events, so as to maintain economic stability. Additionally, the current webinar format lacks spontaneity and the ability or forum to create social bonds with peers. That said, arguments for and against these aspects are likely to remain [81].

Taken as a whole, when being used as a scientific communication tool, webinars are integrating components of in-person conferences, while having enhanced value due to their innate accessibility and functionality as outlined in this chapter. If the guidance in this chapter and elsewhere facilitate a more rapid adoption of webinars in the medical scientific community, one should expect that they will be fully realized as the prominent scientific communication tool of the future.

References

1. Landhuis E. Scientific literature: information overload. Nature. 2016;535(7612):457–8.
2. Robbins R. STAT's guide to health care conferences disrupted by the coronavirus crisis. 2020. https://www.statnews.com/2020/03/07/stats-guide-health-care-conferences-disrupted-covid-19/. Accessed 22 Jun 2020.
3. Langin K. Climate scientists say no to flying. Science. 2019;364(6441):621.
4. Nathans J, Sterling P. Point of view: how scientists can reduce their carbon footprint. 2016. https://elifesciences.org/articles/15928. Accessed 2 Jun 2020.
5. Philippe H. Less is more: decreasing the number of scientific conferences to promote economic degrowth. Trends Genet. 2008;24(6):265–7.
6. Price M. Scientists discover upsides of virtual meetings. Science. 2020;368(6490):457–8.
7. Kwon D. After conference cancellations, some scientists find a way 2020. https://www.the-scientist.com/news-opinion/after-conference-cancellations-some-scientists-find-a-way-67310. Accessed 9 Jun 2020.
8. Fiske P. Why scientists need to market themselves. Nature. 2018;555:7695.
9. Google Scholar. Google. 2020. https://scholar.google.ca/. Accessed 14 Jun 2020.
10. Mendeley Ltd. Mendley. 2020. https://www.mendeley.com/. Accessed 14 Jun 2020.
11. National Center for Biotechnology Information (NCBI). National Library of Medicine (US), National Center for Biotechnology Information, Bethesda. 1988. https://www.ncbi.nlm.nih.gov/genbank/. Accessed 14 Jun 2020.
12. GitHub Inc. GitHub. 2020. https://github.com/. Accessed 14 Jun 2020.
13. Nester R. Webinar and webcast market: global demand, growth analysis & opportunity outlook 2023. 2020. https://www.researchnester.com/reports/webinar-and-webcast-market-global-demand-growth-analysis-opportunity-outlook-2023/237. Accessed 2 Jun 2020.
14. Gerritsen D, Olderen R. Events as a strategic marketing tool. 2nd ed. Wallingford: CABI; 2014.
15. Labagh D. How facebook live connector expands dh webinars. 2020. https://www.on24.com/blog/how-facebook-live-connector-expands-dh-webinars/. Accessed 11 Jun 2020.
16. Feyen EH, Utz RJ, Zuccardi Huertas IE, Bogdan O, Moon J. Macro-financial aspects of climate change. Washington: World Bank Group; 2020.
17. Bosello F, Roson R, Tol RS. Economy-wide estimates of the implications of climate change: human health. Ecol Econ. 2006;58(3):579–91.
18. Mehrabi Z. Food system collapse. Nat Clim Chang. 2020;10(1):16–7.
19. Sarabipour S, Schwessinger B, Mumoki FN, Mwakilili AD, Khan A, Debat HJ, et al. Evaluating features of scientific conferences: a call for improvements. BioRxiv, 2020. https://doi.org/10.1101/2020.04.02.022079.
20. Cisco. Webex, 2020. https://www.webex.com/. Accessed 11 Jun 2020.
21. LogMeIn Inc. Webinar and online conference software. 2020. https://www.gotomeeting.com/en-ca/webinar. Accessed 11 Jun 2020.
22. Association for Medical Education in Europe. Webinars. 2020. https://amee.org/webinars/forthcoming-webinars. Accessed 11 Jun 2020.
23. Honeycomb Worldwide Inc. Upcoming webinars. 2020. https://xtalks.com/webinars/. Accessed 11 Jun 2020.

24. University of Essex. Talks and Tasters. 2020. https://www.essex.ac.uk/visit-us/cant-visit-us/talks-and-tasters. Accessed 11 Jun 2020.
25. Honeycomb Worldewide Inc. Host a webinar. 2020. https://xtalks.com/host-a-webinar/. Accessed 11 Jun 2020.
26. Nagy G. 10 of the best webinar invitation email examples you've ever seen. 2020. https://chamaileon.io/resources/webinar-invitation-email/. Accessed 12 Jun 2020.
27. LogMeln Inc. How do time zones work with scheduling? 2020. https://support.goto.com/webinar/help/how-do-timezones-work-with-scheduling-g2w090102. Accessed 12 Jun 2020.
28. PlusThis. Send sms reminders before your webinar. 2020. https://www.plusthis.com/about. Accessed 12 Jun 2020.
29. Moz Inc. The beginner's guide to seo. 2020. https://moz.com/beginners-guide-to-seo. Accessed 12 Jun 2020.
30. Moz Inc. Backlinks. 2020. https://moz.com/learn/seo/backlinks. Accessed 12 Jun 2020.
31. Cooper P. How the instagram algorithm works in 2020 (and how to work with it). 2020. https://blog.hootsuite.com/instagram-algorithm/. Accessed 12 Jun 2020.
32. van Noorden R. Online collaboration: scientists and the social network. Nature News. 2014;512(7513):126.
33. Buffer. Buffer: Simpler social media tools for authentic engagement. 2020. https://buffer.com/. Accessed 12 Jun 2020.
34. Hootsuite Inc. Hootsuite: social media marketing & management dashboard. 2020. https://hootsuite.com/. Accessed 12 Jun 2020.
35. Ventola CL. Social media and health care professionals: benefits, risks, and best practices. Pharm Therapeut. 2014;39(7):491.
36. Smith K. Invite a colleague to attend—refined support center. 2017. http://support.refineddata.com/hc/en-us/articles/203568390-Invite-a-Colleague-to-Attend-. Accessed 12 Jun 2020.
37. LogMeln Inc. Invite others to join (desktop app)—support. 2020. https://support.goto.com/webinar/help/invite-others-to-join-g2w040002. Accessed 12 Jun 2020.
38. Smith B. How to max out your next webinar with facebook ads. 2016. https://adespresso.com/blog/max-next-webinar-facebook-ads/. Accessed 12 Jun 2020.
39. Capetola T. Drive more webinar registrations with solid ppc campaign management. 2017. https://learn.demio.com/webinar-ppc-campaign-management/. Accessed 12 Jun 2020.
40. Siu E. 54 alternative ad networks to open up new channels of growth in 2020. 2020. https://www.singlegrain.com/blog-posts/pay-per-click/alternative-ad-networks/. Accessed 12 Jun 2020.
41. BigMarker. What's in a webinar title? How to ensure your webinar makes a good first impression. 2017. https://medium.com/@BigMarker/whats-in-a-webinar-title-how-to-ensure-your-webinar-makes-a-good-first-impression-c9d446f95e12. Accessed 12 Jun 2020.
42. LinkedIn Corporation. Making your website shareable on linkedIn. 2017. https://www.linkedin.com/help/linkedin/answer/46687/making-your-website-shareable-on-linkedin?lang=en. Accessed 12 Jun 2020.
43. Shaikh S. The eight secrets to our best webinars. 2019. https://xtalks.com/the-8-secrets-to-our-best-webinars/. Accessed 12 Jun 2020.
44. Winniewong. Google's title and meta descriptions length (Updated 2020). 2020. https://seopressor.com/blog/google-title-meta-descriptions-length/. Accessed 12 Jun 2020.
45. Juurinen A. We analyzed over 100 webinars for title and abstract length: here's how they affect registration rate. 2019. https://xtalks.com/we-analyzed-over-100-webinars-for-title-and-abstract-length-heres-how-they-affect-registration-rate/. Accessed 6 Jun 2020.
46. Parent A. Character limits for paid ads - finally all in one place! 2016. https://www.linkedin.com/pulse/character-limits-paid-ads-finally-all-one-place-alex-parent/. Accessed 12 Jun 2020.
47. Drewitz D. How to write an abstract for your conference talk or webinar. 2019. https://medium.com/@dormaindrewitz/how-to-write-an-abstract-for-your-conference-talk-or-webinar-66ae959be2e6. Accessed 6 Jun 2020.
48. van de Rakt M. Text length: how long should a post or page be? 2020. https://yoast.com/text-length/. Accessed 12 Jun 2020.

49. Baker J. 7 search ranking factors analyzed: a follow-up study. 2018. https://moz.com/blog/7-search-ranking-factors-analyzed-follow-up-study. Accessed 6 Jun 2020.
50. Lloyd-Martin H. What's the 'best' word count for google? [updated for 2019]. 2019. https://seocopywriting.com/whats-the-best-word-count-for-seo-copywriting/. Accessed 6 Jun 2020.
51. Xerox Corporation. 20 ways to share color knowledge. 2017. https://www.office.xerox.com/latest/COLFS-02UA.PDF. Accessed 6 Jun 2020.
52. Lindgaard G, Fernandes G, Dudek C, Brown J. Attention web designers: you have 50 milliseconds to make a good first impression! Behav Inform Technol. 2006;25(2):115–26.
53. Fogg BJ, Soohoo C, Danielson DR, Marable L, Stanford J, Tauber ER. How do users evaluate the credibility of Web sites?. Proceedings of the 2003 conference on designing for user experiences 2003.
54. Gillett R. Why we're more likely to remember content with images and video (infographic). 2014. https://www.fastcompany.com/3035856/why-were-more-likely-to-remember-content-with-images-and-video-infogr. Accessed 6 Jun 2020.
55. Falconer G. The insider's guide to better webinars. 2017. https://logmeincdn.azureedge.net/gotomeetingmedia/-/media/pdfs/gotowebinar-insiders-guide-to-better-webinars.pdf. Accessed 6 Jun 2020.
56. Waechter FM. How to increase conference attendance. 2019. https://congrex.com/blog/how-to-increase-conference-attendance/. Accessed 6 Jun 2020.
57. Springer Nature Limited. Eliminating hiv: bringing together prevention, treatment and cure. 2015. https://www.nature.com/collections/qdtpvmnnqj/webinar. Accessed 12 Jun 2020.
58. McKesson Medical-Surgical. Is your facility secure? Covid-19 issues and beyond. 2020. https://info.mms-ec.mckesson.com/EC_Webinar_20200610_Registration.html. Accessed 12 Jun 2020.
59. Zarrella D. Which types of form fields lower landing page conversions? 2017. https://blog.hubspot.com/blog/tabid/6307/bid/6746/Which-Types-of-Form-Fields-Lower-Landing-Page-Conversions.aspx. Accessed 12 Jun 2020.
60. LogMeIn Inc. Customize emails for webinar event registrants. 2020. https://support.goto.com/webinar/help/customize-emails-for-webinar-registrants-g2w110012. Accessed 12 Jun 2020.
61. State of California Department of Juistice. California consumer privacy act. 2020. https://oag.ca.gov/privacy/ccpa. Accessed 13 Jun 2020.
62. Information Commissioner's Office. Guide to the general data protection regulation. 2020. https://ico.org.uk/for-organisations/guide-to-data-protection/guide-to-the-general-data-protection-regulation-gdpr/. Accessed 13 Jun 2020.
63. Sai. How do I start my event? 2020. https://docs.crowdcast.io/en/articles/768-how-do-i-start-my-event. Accessed 13 Jun 2020.
64. BrightTalk. How do I add my slide presentation into the webinar? 2019. https://support.brighttalk.com/hc/en-us/articles/204280980-How-do-I-add-my-slide-presentation-into-the-webinar. Accessed 13 Jun 2020.
65. Cooley B. Ultimate webcam tips: how to look and sound great online. 2020. https://www.cnet.com/how-to/ultimate-webcam-tips-how-to-look-sound-great-online/. Accessed 5 Jun 2020.
66. Sumby WH, Pollack I. Visual contribution to speech intelligibility in noise. J Acoust Soc Am. 1954;26(2):212–5.
67. Guichon N, Cohen C. The impact of the webcam on an online L2 interaction. Can Modern Lang Rev. 2014;70(3):331–54.
68. LogMeIn Inc. Share handouts during webinars. 2020. https://support.goto.com/webinar/help/share-handouts-during-webinars-g2w020025. Accessed 13 Jun 2020.
69. Minhas PS, Ghosh A, Swanzy L. The effects of passive and active learning on student preference and performance in an undergraduate basic science course. Anat Sci Educ. 2012;5(4):200–7.
70. Zoom Video Communications Inc. Using webinar chat. 2020. https://support.zoom.us/hc/en-us/articles/205761999-Using-webinar-chat. Accessed 13 Jun 2020.
71. Cisco. Generate reports for cisco webex events. 2020. https://help.webex.com/en-us/b7bpy0/Generate-Reports-for-Cisco-Webex-Events. Accessed 13 Jun 2020.

72. Cisco. Create a post-event survey and Add it to an event. 2020. https://help.webex.com/en-us/nbet0py/Create-a-Post-Event-Survey-and-Add-it-to-an-Event. Accessed 13 Jun 2020.
73. On24. Engagement score. 2014. https://communications.on24.com/rs/on24inc/images/ON24_Engagement_Score_Datasheet-A3FD.pdf. Accessed 13 Jun 2020.
74. Anderson C, Duarte N. How to give a killer presentation. Harv Bus Rev. 2013;91(6):121–5.
75. Chapin D. Making the complex compelling: creating high-performance Marketing in the Life Sciences. Nashville: Rockbench Publishing; 2014.
76. Juurinen A. Customer-centric marketing: how to build a strategy for your webinars. 2018. https://xtalks.com/customer-centric-marketing-how-to-build-a-strategy-for-your-webinars/. Accessed 7 Jun 2020.
77. Duarte N. HBR guide to persuasive presentations. Harvard: Harvard Business Press; 2012.
78. Gallo C, Demeda M. The presentation secrets of Steve jobs: how to be insanely great in front of any audience. New York: McGraw-Hill; 2010.
79. Sorensen K. How should I pace my powerpoint presentation? 2020. https://study.com/academy/lesson/how-should-i-pace-my-powerpoint-presentation.html. Accessed 7 Jun 2020.
80. Wolfe A. How to choose the best format for your presentation. 2020. https://blog.polleverywhere.com/presentation-format/. Accessed 7 Jun 2020.
81. Miller A. In some disciplines, heavy drinking is part of the culture. That can be a problem 2018. https://www.sciencemag.org/careers/2018/12/some-disciplines-heavy-drinking-part-culture-can-be-problem. Accessed 13 Jun 2020.

Chapter 11
Just in Time Medical Storytelling

Roger Carl Schank

I had returned to New York from a trip to the UK feeling very badly. I was guessing that I had a kidney stone, but I had had those before and this seemed different. I didn't have a doctor in New York, but a friend told me he could get someone to see me immediately. I saw him and then I got a call from him telling me I was very sick and I needed to see a kidney doctor right away. He set up the appointment for next day. The kidney doctor examined me and told me that I was dying of kidney failure.

Needless to say, I was upset.

His nurse came in and asked me what the kidney doctor (who was listed as one of the top 100 doctors in New York by the way) had said. I told her and she said she had seen a lot of patients who were dying of kidney failure and I didn't look like them at all.

The doctor gave me a diet to follow which he said might help. I started it only to realize that it pretty much described how I normally ate. I returned to Florida getting sicker every day. Finally I called a wealthy friend who had a "concierge doctor" who agreed to see me. The doctor told me to get on the next plane to New York and go to Columbia Presbyterian.

I went and met a kidney doctor there who did something very strange—he listened. He asked me about every detail of my time in the UK and in New York and then told me that I was not dying of kidney failure. He said I had a very high creatinine number which confused the other doctor because it is strongly associated with kidney failure, but what had actually happened to me was that both kidneys were blocked, one by a kidney stone and one because I had managed to dehydrate myself which caused a perfect storm. "Remove the kidney stone and you'll be fine" he said, and they did and I was, and still am 6 years later.

R. C. Schank (✉)
Trump University, New York, NY, USA
e-mail: roger@socraticarts.com

G. C. Di Renzo (ed.), *Essential Writing, Communication and Narrative Skills for Medical Scientists Before and After the COVID Era*,
https://doi.org/10.1007/978-3-030-84954-2_11

Why am I telling this story?

Today we hear endlessly about AI and especially about AI and medicine.

One consistent problem with reporting on AI is that they say AI when they mean "a statistical algorithm." Computer programs can be written to examine reams of data more easily than a person can. This a good thing. But data is easily misunderstood by people (especially when they don't understand the context), and you can be sure these "AI's" won't have a clue. The first kidney doctor I saw looked at a creatinine number over 5 and simply went no further. The nurse looked at me and compared me to other patients she had seen. The Columbia kidney doctor listened and used his vast knowledge of prior cases to reason from.

Modern medicine is full of doctors who are already robotic. But good medicine is like any other subject that requires one to make judgments based on prior cases. You can follow rules, or you can think. The first kidney doctor (who I saw multiple times) never bothered to actually think.

Years ago, in the last AI BS movement of the 1980s, rule-based systems were all the rage. Doctors were interviewed and rules were extracted from them and then computers were given these rules. Suddenly there would be "expert systems," and they would rule the world. VC's dove in head first.

I responded to this expert system nonsense with the idea of case-based reasoning. I said that people reason from past experience, and they do not use rules. (A doctor can glibly give you a rule when asked, but that doesn't mean that they use that rule in decision-making. People are notoriously bad at understanding how their own minds work.)

You want a doctor who has seen a lot of cases similar to yours and can do what that nurse did: recognize something by really looking at the patient. The rule-based systems that caused the AI winter of the 1980s and early 1990s were promising to do something that people don't do: to reason from rules. Now, modern day "AI" is proposing that it can reason from massive amounts of data that the computer really doesn't understand (just like my *NYC Top Doctor* did).

Case-based reasoning proposes that people store and index cases based on many factors and then get reminded of old cases when various factors partially match. Then, and this is the important part, they think about the prior cases more deeply and try to draw the lessons that they learned from the earlier cases to reason from.

We had some success at building case-based reasoning programs and many others are still doing that, but when the funding dried up, this became more difficult. This loss has been magnified by the current "AI" which has no way of reasoning from experience and can only promise conclusions based on data it really doesn't understand. The current AI and medical programs would have had me dying as well.

Dr. Radhakrishnan did something very weird. He asked and he listened carefully to my answers. Until computers can do that they will not replace human doctors (or anyone else who needs to think actually.)

Now, of course, I believe in AI. I worked in it my whole life. But the current AI fad promoted by the media and backed by VC's can only lead to the very thing that people are afraid of: dumb computers replacing thinking people. What should we do?

When videotape equipment became easy to own and use, many large companies began taping their experts. They figured that they could preserve their corporate memory in that way. Today, in all the cases that I know about, those tapes lie on a shelf somewhere. No one ever looks at them. What went wrong?

The main problem was that television confused the makers of these videos. They were all done as if they were doing an hour-long TV show with an interviewer asking questions and the interviewee looking at the interviewer and responding. Whether this makes good hour long television I cannot say, but this is not how people talk to each other. You would never sit down and give a one-hour monologue to someone who was asking your advice (or if you did, you'd soon find you had an extremely bored and fidgety audience). Instead, people communicate by exchanging stories.

Stories come in all shapes and sizes, but each of us has hundreds of personal stories that we tell all the time. To make it clear what I mean by a personal story, here is one of mine.

> It was 1971. I was giving a talk at a conference being held at NYU. I had been a professor at Stanford for two years by this point and had given many such talks in the previous few years, but this one was different. This was my first speech in New York. And, my mother was coming.
>
> She had probably never been to NYU despite having lived in New York City all her life and she certainly hadn't ever been to an academic conference. There weren't many conferences in the bead import business after all. She was coming to see her only child perform and she had dressed for the occasion. She was also fashionably late.
>
> So, somewhere after my speech began, to an audience of shabbily dressed young computer scientists, a middle aged woman entered the lecture hall and took a center seat, causing a row of people to get up as she found her way in. She was dressed in a mink coat and wore pearls. She was clearly noticed by all.
>
> I can't say that I was particularly embarrassed. By the age of 25, I was used to my mother, and I was glad to see she had made it to my talk.
>
> At the end of the speech, after the questions from the audience, she gave me a kiss. I asked her what she thought. She replied that "it was worth every penny."

Now this story is incomplete in the sense that it leaves the listener wondering about several things. What money was my mother talking about, for example?

One of the listeners in my hypothetical room might simply ask that question, and I might respond with another story, possibly longer, where I might explain what my mother meant, how she made me go to college, and why I never took college seriously. By the time I finished my story, the other people in the room would be pretty tired of hearing about me, and more importantly they would all have stories they wanted to tell. What would their stories be about?

One thing we know for sure, because there are unwritten conversational rules about this, and because the human mind works in a very particular way, is that the topics of the stories the rest of the people in the room would tell would be very likely to cover the following terrain:

Their parent's reaction to seeing them for the first time in a professional role.

The embarrassment they might have suffered by having a parent show up in place he or she didn't quite belong.

The first time they gave a professional talk.

Their first day at college.

The right age to start college.

Decisions about which college to attend.

How seriously they took college.

Those are just a few of the possibilities. People have stories to tell about their own lives, they like telling them, and they are reminded of their own stories by other people's stories.

Reminding depends on non-conscious indexing. The seven things I listed above are parts of indices the mind uses to label stories in order to find them again. These labels are not story titles, but a combination of goals, plans, emotions, situations, and typical life decisions that help us understand each other by bringing our own personal knowledge about our lives to bear in order to help us understand the lives of others.

Now imagine if this were an automated intelligent process available on your iPhone. I realize that is a weird idea but not only is this possible it will be available to people soon enough.

The really weird thing about this idea is that the people you would be talking with in this way would be your friends. This seems to work for Facebook in the way that it does, but they are not going out and capturing all of your friends' stories so that they can appear on Facebook when you need them to be there. Maybe someday they will do that.

But, what is more likely, and what is possible right now, is the gathering of expert's stories, in video, and transmitting them to a user just in time when that user needs to hear them.

Here is one such situation. Imagine that you are having a medical problem. You talk about that problem with your friends and they talk about similar situations they themselves have had. People do that all the time. It is not always helpful. Your friends may not know that much.

Or, your "friends" might be professionals in the medical field. They might be the best doctors in the world for example. You should be so lucky.

Well, now you can be that lucky.

We have built a program called EXTRA (Experts telling relevant advice.) EXTRA can be built for any field of expertise where getting the best possible advice in the form of a story told by an expert just in time is a possibility. Medical EXTRA contains (1000 at the time of writing this) stories told by the best and the brightest in medicine. The idea is that a user can be better informed immediately about any problem he might have or be wondering about, as if the best doctors were all the user's best friends, ready to talk at any moment.

These stories are all on video in 1.5 minute clips. They are meant to appear on your computer when the computer "thinks" you need them. As an example here are two (from the same cardiologist):

About 2 months ago, I met a guy for a first time who is 55 years old, a jogger and who has a family history of coronary heart disease but he himself had no known problems. His cholesterol numbers on view were borderline; his blood pressure was normal. But he noticed that he was having some fatigue. And he really didn't *appreciate* any chest pains but he noticed that when he climbed two flights of stairs, he was a little bit more breathy than he used to be and that he stopped walking to work like he use to do, started taking a cab and he just had a sense that something was wrong. Reviewing the symptoms with him and his risk profile his father had a heart attack at a young age, I did a stress test. And he showed severe abnormalities of the stress test suggesting high degree blocking of his coronary arteries. In fact, he had a blockage of 80% of his main artery to his heart. So we recommended fairly urgent bypass. He didn't have chest pains but he definitely knew something was wrong, and he noticed his exercise capacity wasn't as good as it normally is and that he was unconsciously making decisions about limiting his exercise because he just felt something was wrong.

Just last week there was a young man having some chest pain symptoms and he thought he strained a muscle and he spoke to his wife about it and she said look this doesn't sound right and rushed him to the emergency room. And when he came to the emergency room, he had an EKG which is the measuring of the electricity in his heart, and it was clearly showing he was having a heart attack. So nowadays, our hospitals and many like it around the county when that happens we rush in from home. Like this case, I came in from home at 2:00 am in the morning no traffic because it was 2:00 am in the morning and he had a blocked heart artery and by going in through the wrist in his hand and I was actually able to open up his blockage I put a balloon to open it up and then sucked out some clot as well put a stent in there and aborted the heart attack. We did a test on his heart the next day to see how it was functioning, and it was functioning back to normal again. There was no damage at all. Left the hospital 2–3 days later. Two days later and then came to see me after that. He's doing great but the reason this happened is because his wife told him this isn't right and you need to get to the hospital.

We would like computers to be able to tell these stories to the right person at the right time. But is not that so easy.

11.1 Can Computers Tell Stories?

For many years, there has been a dream, held by Artificial Intelligence researchers and others, of a conversational computer, one where a natural dialogue is the means of communication. This dream was subverted by Google in the sense that Google's success at responding to an input of keywords makes users think that they are having a conversation with a computer. Often Google users type in complete English sentences because Google has made them feel as if it is indeed a conversational machine. The fact that the conversation is bizarre from a human point of view doesn't seem to matter. No one asks a friend a question and is happy when he gets back 1000 search results any one of which might or might not answer his question. And certainly no one is happy that for the next question he might have, the computer in no way remembers the context set up by the last one.

So, computers have never really been conversational devices. But what if they were? What do we know about human conversation that would inform us about how to design a conversational computer?

I will take as an example a typical cocktail party conversation between two people who have just met. Here are some rules that participants in such a conversation typically follow:

1. They take turns: one talks for a while, and then the other talks.
2. A speaker must answer a question posed by the other speaker.
3. If there is no question to respond to, the next speaker must say something that relates in some way to what the last speaker has said.
4. Responses must either make the same point ("Something like that happened to me") or make an opposing point ("No, it's not that way, it's this way") or else they must match if no point has been made at all ("Your wife likes to do this, well my wife likes to do this other thing.")
5. Responses cannot be too long. If the intended response is estimated to be more than 2 min long, the speaker must warn the listener in some way ("This may take a little explanation...")
6. Responses are in the form of previously told stories, ones that the speaker has told many time before and one that can be told quickly and efficiently.
7. A story must have a point. If it does not have a point, it must be a no-complex response to the previous remark.

Considering the above rules, rules that are known implicitly by all adult speakers, it is clear why computers are not good conversationalists:

1. Computers have no stories to tell.
2. Computers do not understand the stories being told to them.
3. Even if they did understand the stories being told to them, computers would have no way of matching the points of those stories to the points of the stories they might be able to tell.

The first point is a little strange. Computers do have stories to tell in the sense that any Wikipedia article or New York Times article is a story to which the computer has access. But, the computer doesn't know the stories it has. It can find them through key words and statistics but when it retrieves a story it isn't exactly telling it because it has no idea what it has just said. How could we change this?

11.2 First We Would Need to Give the Computer Stories to Tell

People tell stories in a variety of ways. Novels, newspapers, movies, and TV shows are types of stories. But people have always held one kind of story (the one they were just reminded to tell) as the real thing: the face-to-face spoken story. Our conversations use this normal everyday notion of personal story so often during our daily lives that we often fail to notice its significance. If we were to give computers stories to tell, they would naturally have to start with these kinds of stories. Most of the wisdom that any individual possesses is contained in the form of these kinds of personal stories. Typically such stories are funny or emotional or interesting in some way, and they almost always serve to define some important piece of knowledge or experience of the teller.

And not only do people like to tell personal stories, people like to hear them as well, particularly when a story addresses a problem the listener has and is short and to the point. So the first step in providing computers with stories (not the computer's own personal stories of course) to tell is to record experts telling their personal stories, ones that make a clear point in an interesting way. These should be told with the expert facing the camera directly so that he seems to be in a conversation with the user. And, after the expert's story has been heard, it the computer should be able to offer more personal stories from other experts in order to continue the conversation.

Building such a conversational video story database requires a massive effort at interviewing, collecting, and editing the stories of experts. If the finished system has a few hundred stories in it, it will not be able to sustain an interesting conversation about multiple topics nor will it be able to express multiple points of view. The finished system must be able to surprise the user and must have a great range of wisdom available. This requires thousands of stories.

11.3 The Next Issue in Getting a Computer to Tell Stories Is Retrieval

The computer must be able to retrieve stories by some means other than keywords in order for it to carry on something more closely resembling the way people actually communicate. The way to do this is via indexing.

Every story collected must be indexed; indexing is the trick to making such a system work properly, and it is the intelligence in the system.[1] The indexing cannot be according to keywords, or combinations of keywords, nor can it be alphabetical, organized by speaker, or topic, or any other of the standard indexing schemes that

[1] I first described this in Dynamic Memory (Cambridge Univ Press, 1981)

have been in use for years for books and articles. The indexing scheme must be the one that has been in use for millennia, namely, the one that humans use,

non-consciously, to store and find stories in their own minds with no obvious effort. The index must be identical to what a person would have done when they exclaim after hearing someone say something: *that reminds me of a story!*

What indexing scheme do people use? We can learn about human indexing by looking at how reminding works. When people get reminded of a story by something someone has just said, it is because there is a match between how they indexed what they heard and how they had previously indexed the story they now intend to tell.

We can gain insight into what these indices look like by examining how any story one is reminded of matches an incoming story. We have worked on this problem for years and the answer is that people non-consciously attempt to determine certain the answer to certain questions whenever they are listening to each other. These questions include:

1. What is the actor trying to accomplish?
2. What method is he using to accomplish it?
3. What might be preventing his accomplishing it?
4. What do we know about the particular circumstances?
5. What wisdom is he sharing about what happened?
6. Is there are lesson to be learned from what happened?

As listeners, we don't necessarily realize we are asking these questions. As retrievers of knowledge from own our memory, we don't realize that we use the answers previously generated to these questions as a way of labeling what we have previously experienced. But this is how it happens.

11.4 The Final Issue Involves Giving Computers the Ability to Know When a Situation Warrants the Telling of One Its Stories (and Which One)

In order to make computers into conversational devices that can retrieve stories from a properly indexed memory, the computer must be capable of using the index to make full or partial matches with other stories indexed in the same or similar ways.

A corporate memory, consisting of the experts in a company recalling their experiences, could be used to help people make decisions. But these stories would need to be available at exactly the time the company was making a similar decision. This means that, in essence, the stories from the corporate memory would find you because it knew what you were doing. This is the very opposite of search.

In order for stories to find you, the computer must know who you are and what you are doing. Therefore, a user must be able to make it clear to the computer who he is, what he is doing at the moment, and what his concerns are, in the same language or in some method that uses the same language, that the indexing scheme employed by the computer uses.

When we tell a story to a friend, we know where that friend is, we know what his concerns are, we know is doing in life, and we know what stories we have already told him. We choose to tell a story because we understand that this listener might benefit from it, according to the model we have constructed of that listener. To be useful to people, the computer also needs to know to whom it is speaking. When Expedia or any other travel site suggests flights to me, it acts as if it knows nothing about me and assumes that my biggest concern is the airfare (since it orders possible flights by price). But it could know a lot about me and propose flights according to my concerns which are more about seat comfort and food and ease of transfer, than they are about price.

Viewing flight possibilities as yet another kind of story, Expedia could choose to tell a story that is relevant to me. But this would involve a different kind of technology than the search-based one that we have gotten used to. The next generation of storytelling computers will not only have stories to tell, but also they will also have to know who they are talking to and have a idea about what stories that user already knows. In other words, a conversation-based machine would behave very differently than a search-based machine.

11.5 EXTRA (Experts Telling Relevant Advice)

We have done everything described above in EXTRA, a program that uses cognitive indexing to retrieve stories just in time. These stories can find a user who needs them if it knows what that user is doing. EXTRA can also serve as a system that a user can navigate conversationally to find stories of interest.

The computer's job in EXTRA is to easily integrate new stories and self-organize its memory to make those new stories available. It is not a static system. Its intelligence is in the indexing and in its conception of matching within the indexing. Whenever you hear a story in EXTRA, EXTRA is searching to find one or more related stories to present next.

EXTRA gets smarter over time. Each story it receives is entered into memory and automatically connected to similar stories. The role of the human indexer in EXTRA is simply to index each new story in isolation. EXTRA does the rest.

This allows the creation of a true alternative to keyword based search. Stories are searched for by their conversational relevance which is measured by the closeness of fit of their indices

EXTRA is meant to capture the corporate memory of any large organization with experts who rarely meet each other or who may retire or quit. It is an Artificial Intelligence program in the truest sense of that term. EXTRA is attempting to replicate a human thinking process, one that is somewhat hidden to people but one that use every time they get reminded of something to say and feel the need to say it.

We have been building just in time advisors based on the unconscious reminding process. We start with story collection in a particular domain of knowledge. Stories are then indexed by hand. When enough stories are collected and indexed, a knowledge base of what smart people know about how to deal with complex situations is available to those who need it. The query process depends upon the relating the structure of the tasks in an organization, to its stories, not key words. We have done this for large corporations, for the military and in medicine.

We want to reach the point where the computer can tell you a story because it knows what you are trying do and it knows it has something relevant to say just as a village elder might have done in day gone by.

Companies or organizations that want to capture their expertise have to agree to provide storytellers (e.g., experts in an organization who can tell stories of success and failure and are willing to tell them on camera). It is a shame that we don't know every interesting story in every domain and aren't capable of telling them just in time. This would very important in medicine.

Epilogue

Communicative Theory at the Time of COVID-19 Pandemic

Throughout the COVID-19 pandemic, we are experimenting novel ways of communication. In particular, this new dramatic scenario has imposed the need of developing effectiveness strategies to give updates, statistics, and scientific-medical evidences and communicate policy decisions everywhere and in shorter time than before.

Science communication has become a common focus of many aspects of academic research and teaching. Anyway, its history has ancient origins. The word "science" itself derives from Latin word "scientia" meaning knowledge. In ancient Greece, this imparting of knowledge took place in public debates and involved masses; this democratization of knowledge led to the down of experimentation and the advancement of philosophy and science. Some years later, scientific knowledge transferred also via written words and often hoarded by the privileged few.

The nineteenth century was a time of great change in science, industry, and also communication. Michael Faraday (1801–1867), scientist and science lecturer, could be considered the "father" of early science communication. Faraday loved to call himself a "philosopher of nature," and he is perhaps the first scientist to ask himself how science can move forward, ignoring the community and how, instead, it can contribute to nurturing a different common sense. His "Christmas Lectures for Children" and "Conferences of Friday Evening" were intended for an heterogeneous audience: from insiders to ordinary people who expected rational answers from science, thus maintaining a "democratic attitude" in communicate and spread knowledge to everyone. Faraday demonstrated an inestimable versatility and ability to reach different targets of population thanks to essential qualities such as having unquenchable curiosity, being an acute discoverer, having a passion for clarity in exposition.

G. C. Di Renzo (ed.), *Essential Writing, Communication and Narrative Skills for Medical Scientists Before and After the COVID Era*,
https://doi.org/10.1007/978-3-030-84954-2

Another extremely modern element of Faraday's figure is found in his great sensitivity toward the relationship between science and technology (between basic research and applied research), a convinced supporter of the importance of both without a priority scale. It looks as a prophetic attitude, if we consider how strongly connected science and technology today are and are configured as two aspects of those advances that have changed daily life. Faraday popularized science to adults and children with profound charism, intuition, and technical versatility and in an almost timeless style.

What would Faraday have thought of the current epochal change in the way of communicating?

Nowadays, we are facing the COVID-19 pandemic with still a scarce knowledge of the pathogen and the infection mechanism, but with an extreme need of worldwide exchange and transmission of information for scientific-medical, social, and economic stability.

Faraday's lessons represent an excellent reference model and could be revised and adapted for current science communication in the era of COVID-19 pandemic. His thought and strategy of communication could be shaped to new technologies, scientific researches methodologies, society components, social groups, communities, and jobs.

The current pandemic imposes restrictions in each field of life, including on the ways to communicate. Worldwide exchange of information is now based on "infomedia" strategies and every form of communication in presence is avoided. Scientific conferences, meetings, research projects, and data sharing between social groups are organized via web modalities. Advantages and disadvantages are invocated on these new ways of science communication, with obviously a great heterogeneity of opinions.

The most frequent questions concern if remote communication is really effective and can it reach all social contexts. The remote communication we are experiencing is highlighting the importance of being able to communicate from one part of the world to another and of transmitting scientific data useful for creating attack strategies against this pandemic. Practical examples are how telemedicine is allowing scientists and researchers from all over the world to discuss the clinical course of infection, the development of therapies, to draw national and international guidelines. The researchers are capable of having a virtual physical existence in other labs. Recent advances in remote surgeries performed by robots under the remote control of surgeons who are not physically present represent the realization of this concept. Thus, remote science communication imposed by the current pandemic are stimulating and facilitating distance-education programs, tele-learning, sharing databases, computer-mediated communication, and multidisciplinary cooperative/collaborative learning aspects.

Web-based telecommunication represent an essential tool not only for target social groups (scientific field, economic field, policy strategy) but also to communicate with general population, to give medical-clinical advices and updates of the ongoing pandemic, to inform about policies and economic choices.

On the other hand, remote communication and use of web to transmit knowledge do not always seem to work optimally and sometimes confusion and failure emerge. Why is remote communication not always effective? Is there perhaps a problem of trust toward those who present the data? Do we absorb the charisma of a speaker behind a webcam in an altered way?

Probably the scientific communication system (and not only) imposed by this health emergency is obviously (and probably physiologically) imperfect because not all worldwide contexts were prepared for receive information through web-based transmission.

Returning to the question of what Faraday would think about the way we have been forced to do in scientific communication, considering his great versatile personality, he would welcome remote communication as the best tool available in this historical moment to use in a "democratic way," i.e., speaking with humbleness, charisma, and in a way accessible to all people. A scientific lecturer with a bright mind, curious, and simple in speaking is able to be effective and believable behind a webcam as in a city square or in a classroom. Undoubtedly, science communications are operating under pressure in this period and more than ever a dissemination of scientific data and updates to the global population are necessary.

Scenarios and places where communication is made may probably change and evolve, but the power and essence of scientific knowledge and its teaching tools remain closely linked to the charisma, transparency, and trust data sharing of a brilliant science lecturer.

Faraday summarized these concepts in the sentences below, demonstrating his communicative anachronistic geniality:

> "A lecturer should appear easy and collected, undaunted and unconcerned"
>
> "Lecturers which really teach will never be popular; lecturers which are popular will never really teach"
>
> Michael Faraday & the Editor…

References

1. Bagnoli F, Livi R. Micheal faraday: a virtuos life dedicated to science. Substantia. 2018;2(1):121–34. https://doi.org/10.13128/Substantia-45.
2. Bagnoli F, Lorini D, Lio P. Modeling social groups, policies and cognitive behaviiour in COVID-19 epidemic phases. Basic scenarios. Substantia. 2020;4(1):914. https://doi.org/10.13128/Substantia-914.
3. Chan HF, Ferguson N, Savage D, et al. Is science able to perform under pressure? Insights from COVID-19. CREMA Working Paper No. 2020-07.
4. Zaer H, Fan W, Orlowski D, et al. A Perspective of international collaboration through web-based telecommunication–inspired by COVID-19 crisis. Front Hum Neurosci. 2020;14:577465.

Printed by Printforce, United Kingdom